Developing Practice Knowledge for Health Professionals

D0886007

For Butterworth-Heinemann:

Commissioning Editor: Heidi Allen
Associate Editor: Robert Edwards
Project Controller: Joannah Duncan
Designer: George Ajayi
Illustration Manager: Bruce Hogarth

Developing Practice Knowledge for Health Professionals

Edited by

Joy Higgs PhD, MHPED, GradDipPhty, BSc
Faculty of Health Sciences, University of Sydney, Australia

Barbara Richardson PhD, MSc, MErgs
School of Occupational Therapy and Physiotherapy, School of Health, University of East Anglia, UK

Madeleine Abrandt Dahlgren PhD
Department of Behavioural Sciences, Linköpings Universitet, Sweden

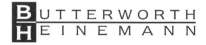

BUTTERWORTH
HEINEMANN

EDINBURGH LONDON NEW YORK OXFORD PHILADELPHIA ST LOUIS SYDNEY TORONTO 2004

BUTTERWORTH-HEINEMANN
An imprint of Elsevier Limited

© 2004, Joy Higgs, Dr Barbara Richardson and
Dr Madeleine Abrandt Dahlgren. All rights reserved.

No part of this publication may be reproduced, stored in a retrieval
system, or transmitted in any form or by any means, electronic,
mechanical, photocopying, recording or otherwise, without either the
prior permission of the publishers or a licence permitting restricted
copying in the United Kingdom issued by the Copyright Licensing
Agency, 90 Tottenham Court Road, London W1T 4LP. Permissions may
be sought directly from Elsevier's Health Sciences Rights Department
in Philadelphia, USA: phone: (+1) 215 238 7869, fax: (+1) 215 238 2239,
e-mail: healthpermissions@elsevier.com. You may also complete
your request on-line via the Elsevier Science homepage
(http://www.elsevier.com), by selecting 'Customer Support' and then
'Obtaining Permissions'.

First published 2004

ISBN 0 7506 5429 5

British Library Cataloguing in Publication Data
A catalogue record for this book is available from the British Library

Library of Congress Cataloging in Publication Data
A catalog record for this book is available from the Library of
Congress

Notice
Medical knowledge is constantly changing. Standard safety precau-
tions must be followed, but as new research and clinical experience
broaden our knowledge, changes in treatment and drug therapy may
become necessary or appropriate. Readers are advised to check the
most current product information provided by the manufacturer of
each drug to be administered to verify the recommended dose, the
method and duration of administration, and contraindications. It is the
responsibility of the practitioner, relying on experience and knowledge
of the patient, to determine dosages and the best treatment for each
individual patient. Neither the Publisher nor the editors assumes any
liability for any injury and/or damage to persons or property arising
from this publication.

The Publisher

your source for books,
journals and multimedia
in the health sciences
www.elsevierhealth.com

The
publisher's
policy is to use
**paper manufactured
from sustainable forests**

Printed in China

Contents

Contributors

Madeleine Abrandt Dahlgren PhD
Department of Behavioural
Sciences
Linköpings Universitet
Linköping
Sweden

Lee Andresen PhD BSc DipEd
Faculty of Health Sciences
University of Sydney
Sydney
Australia

Sarah Beeston BEd DipTP MA
School of Health Sciences
University of East London
London
UK

Ian Edwards PhD BAppScPhysio
GradDipPhysio
School of Health Sciences
University of South Australia
Adelaide
Australia

Della Fish PhD MA MEd DipEd
Kent, Surrey and Sussex
Postgraduate Deanery for
Medical and Dental Education
London
UK

Rob Garbett MSc BN (Hons) RN
Elliot Dynes Rehabilitation Unit
Royal Hospitals Trust, Belfast
Northern Ireland

Bernt Gustavsson PhD
Department of Education
University of Örebro
Örebro
Sweden

Joy Higgs PhD MHPED GradDipPhty BSc
Faculty of Health Sciences
University of Sydney
Sydney
Australia

Mark Jones BS (Psych) GradCert (Physio)
GradDipAdvanManipTher MAppSc
School of Health Sciences
University of South Australia
Adelaide
Australia

Hildur Kalman PT PhD
Department of Philosophy
Faculty of Social Science
University of Tromsø
Tromsø
Norway

Brendan McCormack DPhil BSc (Hons)
Directorate of Education, Research
and Development
Education Centre
Royal Group of Hospitals
Belfast
Northern Ireland

Maeve McGinley BSc(Hons) DipN
CertHSM NDN DipHEContCare
Buncrana
County Donegal
Ireland

Barbara Richardson PhD MSc MErgs
School of Occupational Therapy
and Physiotherapy
School of Health
University of East Anglia
Norwich
UK

Rodd Rothwell BA MA (Psych)
MA (Phil) PhD
School of Behavioural and
Community Health Sciences
University of Sydney
Sydney
Australia

Julius Sim PhD MSc BA
Department of Physiotherapy
Studies

Keele University
Keele
Staffordshire
UK

Björn Sjöström RN PhD
Institute of Health Care Pedagogics
Göteborg University
Göteborg
and
Department of Health Sciences
University of Skövde
Sweden

Dan Stiwne PhD
Department of Behavioural
Sciences
Linköpings Universitet
Linköping
Sweden

Angie Titchen DPhil MSc MCSP
Royal College of Nursing Institute
Oxford
UK
and
Knowledge Centre for Evidence-
Based Practice
Fontys University
Eindhoven
The Netherlands

Preface

The authors of this book have brought their wide range of experience, knowledge and expertise to present many angles of one central argument. We are advocating that practice epistemology, or knowing how practice knowledge is created, used and developed (further), should become an explicit dimension of the core, the regularity and the expectation of professional practice. A clear understanding of epistemological beliefs is especially important in the face of the uncertainties inherent in the information revolution and the postmodern world. *Developing Practice Knowledge for Health Professionals* presents a collection of peer-reviewed chapters which examine four core issues: What constitutes practice knowledge? How is this knowledge created and developed? What are the roles of practitioners, researchers and educators, as individuals and members of their communities of practice, in assisting understanding of and developing practice knowledge? What are the implications of a practice epistemology model for practice, education and research in the health sciences?

We look forward to your participation in this discourse.

Joy Higgs, Barbara Richardson and
Madeleine Abrandt Dahlgren,
2004

Recognising practice epistemology in the health professions

Barbara Richardson, Joy Higgs and
Madeleine Abrandt Dahlgren

INTRODUCTION

In this chapter our aim is to highlight some of the many issues involved in the task of applying and developing professional knowledge in the increasingly diverse settings and groups with which health professionals work within health and social care. We will provide an overview of the processes involved in explaining and generating practice knowledge which are presented in this book and which have implications for professional practice and the capacity of health care professions to retain, strengthen and justify their place in the health care team. First, we make an appraisal of the changing views of health care to help indicate the impact they can have on practice and the importance of having a knowledge of professional practice knowledge today. This is followed by an examination of what we need to know about the different perspectives of knowledge and why we need to be able to recognise the extent of practice knowledge in our practice activities and the ways it is generated. Finally we look at how education, practice and research link together in providing the sources for generating practice knowledge.

An appreciation of the wide variety of sources from which knowledge is generated in professional practice is critical to the development of practice of each individual member of the health professions. Understanding the ways in which different forms of knowledge arise from and become integrated into practice knowledge can help to identify the sources of knowledge which are relevant to the clinical practice, research and education of each profession. This provides a basis for developing a theory of practice knowledge that is an epistemology of practice or practice epistemology. A central tenet of practice epistemology is the recognition of the impact of the setting or situation on the quality, nature and extent of knowledge which is used and generated. Professional knowledge is that which is relevant to and grounded in the practice context. The topic of understanding professional knowledge and the processes of its use and generation has received limited attention in the literature of health professionals to date and yet has become increasingly important to justify practice and practice development. The effects of knowledge which is generated in the practice context need to be more clearly appreciated by teachers, researchers and practitioners alike if the valuable contribution of each health profession is to be fully appreciated and credited in the evolution of health and social care in the 21st century.

CHANGING VIEWS OF HEALTH AND SOCIAL CARE

Understanding practice knowledge and how it is developed is of vital importance to the quality and effectiveness of professional practice in a changing world. Global changes on a number of fronts, including technical, demographic, political and philosophical, have become dominant influences in health and social care. Rapid advances in information technology and communication systems have created an increased communication, via the internet and media coverage, which has helped to broaden our understanding and acceptance of the variety and diversity of lifestyles to which people aspire and to lead to higher levels of health information becoming available, raising public expectations of the standards of health care. Advances in communication systems have also drawn attention to the health status of people globally and highlighted a political and philosophical responsibility of nations to concern themselves with the quality of their people's lives. There is increased emphasis placed upon individuals and their rights to equitable health lifestyles (World Health Organization 1986, 1997).

Many inequalities can be identified in lifestyles today: modern medicine has achieved control of almost all infectious diseases but has not yet managed to halt the development of the chronic diseases which are prevalent in contemporary lifestyles; demographic change to a 'greying' population in most western countries has created an imbalance between the working and retired populations. Concerns for managing the health of ageing populations, with the implied concomitant cost of managing chronic disabilities, have led to economic restraint and political scrutiny of health funding. Such global changes are redefining views on health and illness in the policies and practice of governments and agencies (Neubauer 1998). These changing views of health care will impact greatly on the development of services responsible for people's health and well-being in the 21st century. They will also impact on health professionals themselves as they become confronted by new demands and new expectations of their competence.

The impact of changing views of health care on health professionals

Increasingly the aim of health care is seen to be the provision of support to people in managing their own health and the quality of their lives in their own environments. Health today is thus interpreted more broadly than in the illness remediation goals of much of past medical practice. Today the concept of health encompasses a concern for people's well-being and the quality of their lived experience (Lawson et al 1996). This has led to a concept of health care as being multifaceted. There is a redefinition of the role of patients to consumers of health care with individual goals of wellness which are defined by the links between their health and their ability both to function optimally and to participate fully in their social and occupational activities (World Health Organization 2001). Policy shifts are consequently aimed at providing a market basis for health care which will facilitate delivery of client-focused care through a widening range of services which can match the changing needs of local populations. Cost constraints are prevalent and the pattern of health care is shifting to a decrease in hospital stays and an increase in reliance on self-help at home and support from the community. The increased emphasis on individual rights to high-quality care, together with the dwindling resources available to provide it, have led to demands for cost-effective and evidence-based health practices (Berkman 1996, Muir Gray 1997; Ch. 9). A range of stakeholders (in primary care, long-term care and health promotion as well as in the acute care sector) are increasingly demanding an open accountability of professional work and governance of health care resources. Societal authority and responsibility for health and social care are becoming decentralised and shifted to a local level. As well as achieving the goal of demonstrated accountability, these moves are intended to foster a richness of debate between consumers and purchasers around the commodity of health provided by the health care professions. Professional accountability and governance of health care resources are equally demanded by patients, who have moved from being passive recipients to critical consumers of health. Traditional health care working practices which embodied paternalistic care aimed at eradicating disease are now of necessity being overturned.

The multifaceted nature of health care today presents many challenges in defining, implementing and evaluating practice. A shift has occurred away from medical approaches, which aim to restore people's health to a commonly accepted norm, towards a social model of health care with aims to support the variety of healthy lifestyles which may be desired by individuals. This shift means that the professional task must be opportunistically gleaned and defined, in contexts of care which cannot be fully predicted. The onus will increasingly be on each health professional to take an active and responsible role in defining a professional task in each care context, to identify the health issues and client populations relevant to their profession and to negotiate how to work with them. The increasing move of health care services into community settings calls for practitioners to be creative in problem-solving and to utilise sound analytical skills, not only to design desirable futures for their individual clients, but also to devise ways of working with them to achieve these outcomes (Ackoff 1979, p. 100, cited in Schön 1991, p. 16). Strategies to establish a continuity of interaction with people over long periods of their lives in longitudinal and ambulatory care (Bordage et al 1998) will be key issues for practitioners when planning self-care programmes for individual clients.

These shifts in health care policies offer opportunity for the nature and characteristic structure of health and social care services to be determined both by public and professional advocacy for a health and social care system that is perceived to be cost-effective and relevant to contemporary lifestyles. Each profession needs to be alert to the abundant opportunities and constraints to professional practice development created by these changing aims of health care if they are to ensure that their own professional development and that of their profession will not be restricted in providing high standards of quality in care. This points to a need for all health professionals to develop the capacity to determine their professional responsibility not only towards the single case, but also a capacity to be knowledgeable about the characteristics of their specific profession in relation to other professions and to societal demands. They need to understand and be able to explain the goals and values of their practice and the basis of their professional knowledge.

The importance of knowing the individual characteristics of the knowledge base of your practice

Individual client needs are best revealed and identified through the interactions within the team of health care workers as well as clients themselves. Such collaborative work, supported by a broadening access to health literature for both clients and professionals, can raise the standards of professional care and also the level of public understanding of the possibilities and limitations of that care. There will be an increasing expectation that professional decision-making will be part of a mutual clinician–client process and it will be important for professionals to be able to explain and negotiate openly with their clients and fellow health care workers concerning the services they are able to offer. However, more scrutiny of the specific work (and the underpinning theories) of each profession by clients and other health stakeholders in multidisciplinary, interdisciplinary and transdisciplinary health care teams can constrain emerging techniques and approaches of individual professions and influence the development of their theory and practice (Eakin & Heather 1992). Activities such as clinical audit programmes and critical care pathways, imposed through the management of ever-diminishing health funds, can limit creative and innovative work based on professional judgement, constrain exploration of the modification or development of techniques and raise ethical concerns of care (Ch. 8). Practitioners need to be prepared to evaluate their practice, to critique the evidence they base their practice on and to see themselves as agents of change who are confidently able to defend the work and the quality of care their profession offers. This ability to respond to change and to put forward an explicit rationale for the evidence base of our practice will be critical to our ongoing capacity as an individual to provide quality health care and to maintain a strong professional profile in the health care team and with the public at large.

In 'real world' practice, effective and sustainable change is more likely to be generated bottom-up than top-down by the day-to-day decision-making and working relationships of the players in the field of health care, that is, the therapists, nurses, doctors and their direct managers. The stage has thus been set for systems of working which altruistically can offer great potential for positive changes in health and social care. An emphasis on wellness care of individuals and the critical scrutiny of accountability measures can provide the stimulus for enormous steps forward in the development of health care practice and for each profession to maximise its individual contribution to health care. However, there are many challenges to be addressed if these opportunities are to be seized. This book examines some of the challenges presented in the understanding, explication and valuing of an epistemology of practice. That is, of knowing how we come to know about what we do in practice and being able to identify the individual and the difference in characteristics of our professional knowledge base.

THE NEED FOR A KNOWLEDGE OF KNOWLEDGE

Epistemology is the branch of philosophy that investigates the origins, nature, methods and limits of human knowledge. Practice epistemology refers to the nature of knowledge and the processes of generation of knowledge which underlie practice. We contend that health professionals need a judicious working knowledge of their practice epistemology in order to understand what drives their actions, to realise how they can demonstrate this understanding in their practice and to recognise how they learn from this understanding and develop their professional practice. The responsibility for each profession to explicate and generate professional knowledge which is relevant to contemporary practice is no less demanding than the responsibility for each profession to update and credibly use professional knowledge. At this time, when communities, governments and employers are demanding cost-effective and evidence-based practice, it is important to examine how and why decisions are made within each specific health care event. We need to gain a deep understanding of the nature of the knowledge that underpins our practice in order to create a framework for professional debate which can facilitate optimal practice quality and development. Identifying and describing the extent of our practice knowledge, gaining a knowledge of our knowledge, can help develop our capacity to provide a convincing justification of our professional knowledge which can maintain our unique, viable and valued professional profiles within the range of professions engaged in helping to achieve people's health and well-being.

Recognising dimensions of professional knowledge

Professional knowledge is built upon existing knowledge and upon the conscious and unconscious beliefs and values held by practitioners about what they do, how they do it and why they do it (Chs 3 and 4). The extent to which professional practice is publicly discussed and acknowledged by professionals is influenced by the value the members of a profession place upon several important factors. The first of these is the characteristics and extent of the knowledge which is recognised to comprise the professional knowledge base. The second is the recognition of the dynamic nature of this knowledge base. The third is the acceptance to make credible and appropriate modifications, adaptations and innovations to practice and to practice knowledge in response to changing contexts of care. The problems inherent in the everyday world of practice form a framework for developing knowledge which has its origins in the reality of practitioners' lived experience (Eakin & Heather 1992). However, different beliefs about knowledge and its role in practice can lead to different rules for determining whether this knowledge is accepted as true, real or valid (Pallas 2001) (Ch. 4). Differing beliefs about what counts as knowledge, what counts as evidence for a claim of knowledge, and what counts as a warrant or guarantee for that claim are central in determining what a profession knows about its subject matter (ibid.) (Ch. 6). Development of a profession's knowledge base can be limited if the nature and dimensions of the knowledge underpinning practice are not well understood by the practitioners.

The values which underpin much of the experience of western health care practice today endorse a view of individuals as being unique, endowed with rights of dignity, equality and self-determination, and with functional needs which are relative to their physical, spiritual, cultural and social environment. Nationally and internationally, health needs are being redefined through policy statements and other global declarations of health which encourage approaches to health care that focus upon individuals and their quality of life rather than their disease or disability status (World Health Organization 1986, 1997). The essential needs of individuals to become empowered to maintain a good-quality and healthy lifestyle cannot be generalised but must be negotiated for each person in his or her own setting. The pivotal contribution of artistry in professional judgement is beginning to gain recognition in a new understanding of the concept of clinical effectiveness when dealing with the 'messy' (Schön 1991, p. 16) practice of real-world settings, particularly in primary care, community care and long-term care. The whole area of professional judgement creates a fascinating but problematic paradox. On the one hand, the use of professional knowledge is valued as a basis for making professional judgements in complex situations where there is often no single right answer. On the other hand, the value placed on an evidence-based practice (EBP) currently promulgated in the health care system leads to an overreliance on or expectation of a correct answer or a clear-cut 'best practice'. In this context professional judgements can be unfairly criticised as an overemphasis on subjective views and the affective dimensions of the client's lifestyle preferences and aspirations. Where an extreme view of EBP is adopted, demands for scientific evidence can be validly provided only through research carried out through randomised controlled trials. Such research ignores the individual, concentrating instead on manipulation of variables to provide a generalisation of ideas (Robinson & Norris 2001) (Ch. 9). Under this limited definition of EBP, much client-focused work carried out, by the allied health professions in particular, does not attract the credit it deserves. The value of a breadth of professional knowledge which embraces the difference in perspective and the relationship between expertise and practice-generated knowledge and the important part played by practice wisdom in professional judgement needs to be more appreciated. Practice wisdom refers to the capacity to generate, use and critique a range of different forms of knowledge at high levels of skill in achieving successful outcomes of health and social care interventions (Ch. 6). Such wisdom is vital to quality health care and, particularly, to long-term care and chronic disability management.

Recognising different perspectives of knowledge and different modes of knowledge generation

With regard to the competitive environment of changes in health care and the changes in health focus, the professions are challenged to evaluate and critique their practices, the modes of knowledge generation which lead to development of them, and the way sources of professional knowledge are valued and reflected in goals of practice (Chs 3–5). Professional practice knowledge refers to the knowledge base used by an individual or a profession. It comprises propositional knowledge (knowledge derived from research and theory) and professional craft knowledge (knowledge derived from professional experience) (Higgs et al 2001). Professional practice also utilises personal knowledge (knowledge derived from the personal experience of the individual) (ibid.). Health practitioners are familiar with the acquisition or learning of existing knowledge. Commonly this is regarded as practice knowledge of the field, and this term is particularly used to refer to propositional knowledge and to the technical or procedural aspects of professional craft knowledge. Health professionals are less familiar with the processes involved in the generation of knowledge, which is often mistakenly seen as largely being the province of researchers. Yet practitioners are continually engaged in knowledge generation, particularly through processing and making sense of their professional experiences. Practice wisdom is generated from practice experience when cognitive and metacognitive processes are linked in the clinical reasoning, professional judgements and the affective processes which together produce 'cultural competence' (Engel 2001, p. 17). These processes are the basis of applying professional knowledge in practice situations (Chs 3, 5 and 11).

The generation of practice knowledge thus occurs from practice settings through the world view (or ontological perspective) and the approach to knowing (epistemology) of practitioners themselves. Ontology refers to the framework in which knowledge is generated and recognised. That is, consciously or unconsciously, practice knowledge is founded upon the ontological perspective of practitioners that defines a reality of their practice and their clients which integrally relates their views of knowledge and evidence (Chs 3 and 5). If practice evidence is based largely on an ontological view of people as objects whose deviation from an accepted norm of behaviour can be manipulated and controlled, a full recognition of the experiential contribution to competent and effective practice will be limited. Working with people in the health and social sciences requires a world view which acknowledges a range of values of individuals and their relationships with others and their environment. This emphasises the important influence of the experiential and tacit dimensions of practitioners' knowledge which become amalgamated into their understanding of the wide diversity in people's behaviour and motivations. A tension is thus created between schools of thought which are polarised towards a view of knowledge which is concrete, objective and generalisable and a view of knowledge which is interpretive, subjective and contextual.

The implications to practice of holding differing views of professional knowledge

Knowledge which is viewed as constructed by individuals through interpretation of their context endorses an understanding of the multiple ways in which people perceive reality, and the multiple ways in which the quality of life has meaning for them, as an important tool to assist health professionals in their role of empowering clients to manage and enhance their health. It endorses a concept that people perceive the world in multiple ways through a world view constructed through their individual life experiences.

Recognition of the multiple realities presented by clients acknowledges the powerful symbolism in our lived experience and how it can influence and shape further experiences and interactions. This constructivist view of knowledge embraces a belief that there are many different ways of seeing and existing in the world, and is congruent with the multiplicity of client needs encountered in professional practice today. An understanding of reality as being individually and socially constructed is germane to client-focused practice because it acknowledges a need to work with individuality and variety, and to understand the social contexts of each of our clients. This understanding provides us with a valuable direction for understanding and developing practice. It also gives us confidence to explain our actions in the context of our practice settings, because it places learning from experience in a central position in knowledge development (Ch. 5). Holding a view of people as interactive beings who develop their knowledge of reality as individuals helps us appreciate how the experiential knowledge of professionals can contribute to their expertise (Ch. 11) in guiding choices of action to enable people to move towards their desired goals of health. An acceptance of the central place of experiential knowledge in expertise in this way facilitates an approach to knowledge generation in which knowledge is viewed as a tool of empowerment by individual practitioners or within a profession, which endorses the differences in knowledge bases among professions. This, in turn, offers practitioners a freedom and autonomy to use many forms of knowledge which are appropriate to work towards their practice goals. Until the construction of practice knowledge is more completely understood to include a range of forms of knowledge, the work of many health care workers will not be presented in ways that will attract the value it deserves in an efficacious and cost-effective system of health and social care.

Practitioners who see their practice as a self-determined, dynamic and critically valued process, rather than as a process carried out under constraints imposed by others, will believe more strongly in their ability to influence its evolution. Self-efficacy beliefs can have a powerful effect on the course of actions people take in their life (Bandura 1989) and their professional pathways. The stronger people's self-beliefs in their capabilities, the greater will be their interest in better ways to prepare themselves educationally (ibid.), to expand their knowledge bases and to present their work more clearly to others. Their drive to personal and professional development has implications for practice development (Ch. 7), development of research into practice knowledge (Ch. 10) and the development of clinical reasoning and expertise (Ch. 11). A commitment to lifelong learning and improving competence as a self-directed professional is fundamental to professional knowledge development. A key goal of this book is to provide an explanation of the ways in which professional knowledge is generated and constructed in a continuum of practice knowledge, and the extent to which the interplay of different forms of knowledge underpins the reality of practice and its development. This critical approach to professional knowledge supports reflective practice as a legitimate means of knowledge generation by practitioners for practitioners because it is through reflection on the outcome of their professional judgements that they learn from their experience (Ch. 2). Reflection can serve as an important mode of self-audit for maintaining day-to-day standards of care and as a spur to self-directed learning (Ch. 2). Such critical appraisal for lifelong learning will enhance the practice of individuals and their professions and in this way professional practice incorporates and builds upon practice epistemology. However, the differing views of knowledge in professional practice need to be clearly articulated in order for education to foster an understanding of them and for research to be able to appraise them fully to enlighten further knowledge development.

RECOGNISING THE LINKS BETWEEN PRACTICE, RESEARCH AND EDUCATION IN THE DEVELOPMENT AND GENERATION OF PROFESSIONAL KNOWLEDGE

Health care work is inexact: it is rarely precise or prescriptive, and is carried out dynamically in unpredictable multidisciplinary social groups that are far removed from the controlled rule-dominated environment of the laboratory or the purely physical world. The interactions between the people involved in any health care event can fundamentally influence the realisation of the intervention and the outcomes of the intervention planned by an individual professional. There is rarely an ideal practice strategy which can be agreed as uniquely suitable to be pursued on each occasion of health care. Instead, clinical effectiveness is attained by responding to the situation, using a wide range of knowledge drawn from several sources. The practitioner's awareness of the dynamic nature of the theoretical bases of this diverse body of knowledge is fundamental to embracing the ontological view of human function (World Health Organization 2001) which takes into account the meaning people attach to the behaviour of others and the way this influences their own behaviour. This further legitimises the position that people are self-determining and autonomous, and equally endorses a view of practitioners as able to understand and influence the responses and actions of others with whom they are involved, whether clients or health professionals. Much of this is achieved through the use of reflection on their practice. This is central to developing an understanding of the social structures and the constraining, limiting and enabling influences in health care environments which contribute to the final outcome of their competent care.

Recognising competence in practice

The argument in favour of practitioners being reflective about their practice has influenced the discourse on professional knowledge since the early 1980s, when Schön published his seminal work, *The Reflective Practitioner* (1983, revised 1991). It is now very relevant to extend this discussion into identifying the endeavours which will produce reflective practitioners of the 21st century. We need to identify connections between different modes of reflection in the formation and use of practice knowledge. For instance, metacognition is used within the immediacy of clinical reasoning to critique the choice, use and soundness of knowledge being applied to the clinical problem; reflection-upon-action can be used after clinical decision-making and practice intervention to critique the immediate episode and identify learning outcomes and goals; peer reflection can have value in exposing knowledge claims and emerging ideas to the critical appraisal of others. Reflective thinking which is critical (Maudsley & Strivens 2000) can help us to recognise all the dimensions of professional knowledge that are employed in competent practice.

Professional competence can be regarded as the currency on which the health care market is based. How competence is understood and judged is critical to the employment and deployment of health care workers and to the identification of the needs of professional research and education programmes. In advanced professional practice, the clinician learns to demonstrate professional artistry. This involves using critical thinking as well as intuition, creativity, reflection and lateral thinking to critique, use and develop knowledge in practice. Such clinical expertise relies on tacit knowledge and professional judgements grounded in a depth of professional knowledge and experience, regardless of the field of professional practice. These judgements are made on several levels of practice, as Handal and Lauvås (2000) describe using examples from the professional field of teaching. The action level comprises judgement about what action to take in a specific situation and how it is carried out. The legitimation level involves consideration of how actions are motivated and grounded in the professional knowledge base, which consists of both experiential knowledge and conveyed knowledge from books, research or other sources. At the ethical level, judgements are made regarding the ethical soundness of the actions taken (Ch. 8).

Linking practice to research and education

Talking about these modes of making professional judgements with others can help health professionals map out their practice knowledge and critically evaluate their reasoning. An articulation of this knowledge and reasoning to other disciplines facilitates a mutual education which helps to gain credit and respect for the role each profession can play in health care. Systematically mapping out the dimensions of clinical practice can enhance knowledge of the ways people work and of the contexts in which they work. Shedding light on knowledge sources (research-based and experiential) in practice and on how issues in the workplace are recognised and addressed can identify epistemological needs for research which explores ways to authenticate the various dimensions of practice. An evaluative approach to clinical practice (Ch. 6) can help to actualise and build links between clinical practice and research which can provide a means for developing an evidence base of practice that is relevant to the skills and aspirations of individual professions. For example, community-based practitioners may be challenged by questions of a qualitative nature such as matters associated with the right of individuals to risk living at home independently; the critical issues that arise for them; how they can best be supported by agencies. The scientific or hypothetico-deductive model that underpins the EBP movement can constrain research questions by defining what is known and which questions can be asked (Garvin 2001). This approach gives no credit to the phenomena of personal meaning in the fluidity of subjective experience which people use to make sense of their lives and guide their actions in matters of health care. An understanding of their practice epistemology can have a significant impact upon the capacity of professionals to reflect on the ways they recognise and respond to the changing demands of health care and to advocate strongly for appropriate research which explores how their reflective practice helps them to work more effectively. Since specific answers are needed for specific professions, it is important for clinical practitioners to understand the essential role they play in contributing to the development of the evidence base of their practice (Ch. 9). Knowledge generation strategies (including research) need to be accepted as credible to other professions if the findings are to be incorporated into the health sciences literature.

It is important for clinicians and researchers to appreciate the diversity of the epistemologies of practice, of the values and understanding of knowledge they may encounter in other health care practitioners (Ch. 10). Philosophical and epistemological differences which represent different positions on justifiable reasons for predictability of human behaviour can have a significant influence on the success of research funding applications and on the peer review processes which determine publication of research (Garvin 2001). If professional groups appreciate a need to generate research that can help develop their views of the expanding fields of their practice, they may more ably present it in ways which justify its veracity to other health care professions. A practical understanding of the multiple epistemological perspectives intrinsic to health and social care work settings is important to break down the professional boundary barriers of health care which can lead to collaborative advanced thinking and knowledge production from which clients can genuinely benefit. Much of the success of this mutual understanding is contingent upon education programmes and the professional socialisation of undergraduate and postgraduate health care students, whether as clinicians, educators or researchers (Ch. 5).

The received knowledge of education programmes marks out the procedures of practice of each profession. However, it is individual practitioners' interpretation of the message of education, together with their response to the situational factors of practice, which will determine how the procedural and propositional knowledge learned in an educational setting will be assimilated into clinical practice. Clinical supervisors or mentors play a key role in guiding students to appreciate the way the professional context shapes their understanding of the phenomena of practice, the many sources of experience which guide their behaviour and their decision-making, and how that contributes to the development of professional knowledge. Socialisation processes (Ch. 5) can ensure that students develop a balanced view of the different modes of knowledge used in their work and encourage them to adopt the sceptical attitude, which is necessary for critical thinking for lifelong learning, that belief is accepted tentatively in the context of current available knowledge (Ikuenobe 2001). Recognition of a central principle of human fallibility in practice epistemology (ibid.) can facilitate a freedom for learners as individuals to accommodate to change and purposefully to maintain the generation of professional knowledge which is relevant to their practice. The debate about whether knowledge of the world can be evaluated independently of the social and historical contexts in which it exists, or whether it is contingent upon or relevant to particular circumstances (Pallas 2001), is becoming more pertinent and critical to the developing standards of health and social care. Practitioners can become aware of themselves as agents of change in all aspects of their professional work if the powerful influences on the ways they use and explain essential elements of their professional knowledge can be made more explicit.

SUMMARY

Insights into the foundations on which our practice is based can help us respond to the glare of scrutiny in contemporary health care. The questions of what professional knowledge is, how we realise it through our practice and how we explain the underlying rules have never been more demanding. Revealing the knowledge that underpins practice can liberate us from confines of traditions which have imposed limits on our practice and practice knowledge. It can prevent the 'new limitation' that EBP, in its extreme form with its heavy emphasis on the primacy of scientific knowledge, seeks to impose on practice knowledge. The way practice in health and social care is judged and the criteria upon which these judgements are based will have a significant impact upon the standard of health care globally. The rules of current practice and its inherent ontological perspective will drive health care policy in the 21st century. As set out in this chapter, this book aims to unravel and explicate some of the threads of discourse of professional knowledge. It offers a framework for articulating and justifying the dimensions and scope of knowledge which underpins good practice in health today which can help to ensure that people continue to have the opportunity to receive the benefits of best practice from each health profession.

REFERENCES

Ackoff, R. (1979). The future of operational research is past. *Journal of the Operational Research Society*, **104**, 100.

Bandura, A. (1989). Perceived self-efficacy in the exercise of personal agency. *The Psychologist*, **10**, 411–24.

Berkman, B. (1996). The emerging health care world: implications for social work practice and education. *Social Work: Journal of National Association of Social Workers*, **41**(5), 541–51.

Bordage, G., Burack, J. H., Irby, D. M. & Stritter, F. T. (1998). Education in ambulatory settings: developing valid measures of educational outcomes and other research priorities. *Academic Medicine*, **73**(7), 743–50.

Eakin, J. M. & Heather, M. (1992). A critical perspective on research and knowledge development in health promotion. *Canadian Journal of Public Health*, **83**(suppl. 1), S73–6.

Engel, C. E. (2001). *Towards a European Approach to an Enhanced Education of the Health Professions in the 21st Century*. Report of the European Interprofessional Consultation 1999–2001. London: UK Centre for the Advancement of Interprofessional Education.

Garvin, T. (2001). Analytical paradigms: the epistemological distances between scientists, policy makers and the public. *Risk Analysis*, **21**(3), 443–55.

Handal, G. & Lauvås, P. (2000). *På Egna Villkor: En Strategi för Handledning [On your own Terms: A Strategy for Counseling]*. Lund: Studentlitterature.

Higgs, J., Titchen, A. & Neville, V. (2001). Professional practice and knowledge. In *Practice Knowledge and Expertise in the Health Professions* (J. Higgs & A. Titchen, eds) pp. 3–9. Oxford: Butterworth-Heinemann.

Ikuenobe, P. (2001). Questioning as an epistemic process of critical thinking. *Educational Philosophy and Theory*, **33**(3 & 4), 325–41.

Lawson, J. S., Rotem, A. & Bates, P. W. (1996). *From Clinician to Manager: An Introduction to Hospital and Health Services Management*. Sydney: McGraw Hill.

Maudsley, G. & Strivens, J. (2000). Promoting professional knowledge, experiential learning and critical thinking in medical students. *Medical Education*, **34**, 535–44.

Muir-Gray, J. A. (1997). *Evidence-Based Healthcare: How to Make Health Policy and Management Decisions*. London: Churchill Livingstone.

Neubauer, D. (1998). *Impacts of Globalization on Health and Health Care Policy*. Occasional paper no. 1. Sydney, NSW: Centre for Professional Education Advancement, the University of Sydney.

Pallas, A. M. (2001). Preparing education doctoral students for epistemological discovery. *Educational Researcher*, **30**(5), 6–11.

Robinson, J. E. & Norris, N. F. J. (2001). Generalisation: the linchpin of evidence-based practice? *Educational Action Research*, **9**(2), 303–8.

Schön, D. A. (1991). *The Reflective Practitioner: How Professionals Think in Action*. Aldershot: Arena.

World Health Organization (1986). *Ottawa Charter*. Available at http://www.who.int/hpr/archives/docs/ottawal.

World Health Organization (1997). *Jakarta Declaration*. Available at http://www.who.int/hpr/archive/docs/jakarta.

World Health Organization (2001). *International Classification of Functioning, Disability and Health*. Geneva: WHO. Available at http://www.who.int/icidh.

2

Redefining the reflective practitioner

Madeleine Abrandt Dahlgren,
Barbara Richardson and Hildur Kalman

INTRODUCTION

This chapter outlines the theoretical background that is commonly referred to when we talk about reflecting in practice. Its point of departure is the discussion in the literature of the concepts of *reflective practice, reflective practitioner* and *professional competence* during the last few decades.

The description of the theoretical basis for reflective practice begins with a critique of the use of technical rationality and science as a base for the professions, and proceeds to advocate a focus on situated action and recognition of the pivotal place of the knowledge of the individual practitioner in the synthesis of practice strategies and approaches. Consideration follows of professional competence and how it differs from professional knowledge and other kinds of knowledge. The emphasis is on the need for the development of a practical and discursive consciousness in professionals, reflecting not only *in* or *on*, but also *about* practice, as a condition for shaping the future profession. Subsequently there is discussion of the need for a renewed and critical understanding of the concept of reflective practice. The reflective practitioner of the 21st century must be able to reflect on what is meant by evidence and how professional knowledge is generated. Practitioners also need to be challenged to reflect on and articulate intuitive criteria for judgement to justify knowledge that is generated and resides in the experiential dimension. Further, practitioners need to take responsibility for encouraging articulation of research that can be undertaken to create or further develop the evidence base for practice. The final part of the chapter deals with educational implications concerning fostering reflective practice in the education of health professionals, and how educational strategies can promote or hamper the development of reflective practitioners. The core capabilities needed for reflective practice are delineated.

THE CALL FOR AN ALTERNATIVE EPISTEMOLOGY OF PRACTICE: THE REFLECTIVE PRACTITIONER AND THE NOTION OF REFLECTIVE PRACTICE

The notion of reflective practice has become widely recognised across a range of professions since Donald Schön minted the concept in his books *The Reflective Practitioner* (1983) and *Educating the Reflective Practitioner* (1987). The main point of Schön's argument for an alternative epistemology of practice is that the nature of practice knowledge cannot be described from the viewpoint of the positivist epistemology prevailing in modern universities. The modern research university was derived from the doctrine of positivism, Schön argued, and the universities' business was to produce new scientific and systematic knowledge according to this epistemological view. When professional schools moved into universities in the 1920s they had to conform to the epistemology established in the university and to construe professional knowledge as the application of research (Schön 1987). Schön referred to this perspective of knowledge as technical rationality, arguing that technical rationality is inadequate to describe how professionals think in action.

Critiquing technical rationality

According to a technical rationality position, practical knowledge is the application of universal theories and universal rules. In this view the problems of professional fields are instrumental and professional practice is a process of problem-solving. Problems are solved through selection from available means fitting established ends. This is not, however, how practice presents itself to practitioners. On the contrary, Schön (1987) argued that the practice field is 'messy', problems are ill-defined and knowledgeable practitioners need to read the unique existing situation and to 'set' the problem in order to be able to solve it. The *naming* and *framing* of the problem are important features of the professional's practice knowledge. Problems are not just given or 'out there', they are constructed in interaction with the situation. Instead of universal rules to be applied, professionals have access to a repertoire of examples, images, interpretations and actions that function as metaphors for how the unique situation could be interpreted. Some of these metaphors are conveyed through the discourse and behavioural norms of the professional community of practice, while others are generated from the practitioner's experience. Certainly the practitioner often has access to formal theories and rules, but they are subordinated in the sense that they become actualised only after problem-setting, meaning construction and problem formulation. When practitioners construct meaning for a unique situation, they see it as something that (commonly) already exists in their repertoire.

For experienced and reflective practitioners, we also recognise that these individuals move beyond what already exists in their repertoire to continue to enlarge and refine their repertoires, expanding the range of metaphors and possibilities from which to create the current unique solution. This means that a familiar situation functions as metaphor or pattern for the interpretation of the new situation. Practitioners also choose which action to take according to their situational interpretation, by comparing their previous actions in a familiar situation. From this point of view, knowledge is not manifested in the subjects' minds as a representation of an external world, but exists as a relation between questions and answers in a context of meaning which, in action, leads from task to fulfilment within different human activities (Molander 1993). In describing this picture of practitioners' knowledge and actions we are speaking of practitioners who have had sufficient workplace experience to build up the repertoire of actions and knowledge described. Novices will progressively develop this capability.

Other central features in Schön's writings are the concepts *reflection-in-action* and *reflection-on-action*. With reflection-in-action, the practitioner sets the problem anew when the situation 'talks back': reflection-in-action involves a surprise, a response to surprise as the practitioners think about what they are doing while they are doing it. They are setting the problem of the situation anew, conducting an action experiment on the spot by which they seek to solve the new problems they have set, an experiment in which they test their new way of seeing the situation and also try to change that situation for the better (Schön 1995). Schön's writings about reflection-in-action have been critiqued by, among others, Rolf (1991), who questioned whether it is possible to reflect consciously while engaged in the task or whether reflection-in-action is a process where knowledge functions tacitly and only afterwards can be subjected to reflection, reflection-on-action. Rolf referred to Polanyi's theory (1966) that knowing comprises a tacit dimension that functions as an active shaping of experience and tacitly integrates theoretical and practical knowledge. The important message and conclusion to be drawn from the literature regarding the nature of practice knowledge that we want to acknowledge in this chapter is that tacit knowledge is not to be understood as non-accessible knowledge. It is possible to subject experiences to reflection and thereby construct and reconstruct a considerable part of the clinical reasoning residing in the tacit dimension, even if there might still be parts of our knowing that we cannot access through reflection.

Reflection-on-action refers to the practitioner articulating the processes of the action and the decisions made. It can also involve reflecting on reflection-in-action. Reflection-on-action is regarded as important for enhancing and building the practitioner's knowledge base.

Schön's notion of reflective practice and his concept of the reflective practitioner created a crucial change of perspective about what is understood about practice knowledge. He emphasised situated action and recognised the pivotal place of the unique knowledge base of the individual practitioner in the synthesis of practice strategies and approaches. This had a profound influence on professional educational programmes within a wide range of areas. A number of people have also criticised the manner in which the notion of reflective practice has sometimes been adopted more like a 'mantric theory' than as a true critical stance towards practice (Ball 1994, cited in Ecclestone 1996). The routinised use of various checklists and other devices that are aimed at enhancing reflection in students could turn the reflective act into a mechanised rote-learning activity. The notion of the reflective practitioner has also influenced contemporary discourse about what constitutes professional competence, as is outlined in the following section.

Perspectives on professional competence

Perspectives on professional competence have changed over time. Traditional perspectives, influenced by a theoretical knowledge tradition and the ideals of positivism, take as their point of departure a dualistic perspective of knowledge as a product, transferable from research, through education, into professional practice (Rolf et al 1993). In this framework professional competence is science-based, implying the application of scientific theories to defined problems in the professional practice. According to Sandberg (1994), this scientification of professional practice reflects a dualistic ontology, comprising a division of the phenomenon of competence into two separate entities, the worker and the work. The positivistic epistemology (in this instance referring to an objective, knowable work beyond the worker) has led to descriptions of work activities that are independent of the worker who accomplishes them. Rationalistic approaches thus identify and describe human competence as constituted by two independent entities, a list of attributes possessed by the worker externally related to a list of work activities (ibid).

Svensson (1996) argued similarly that the traditional perspectives on competence could be described as *behaviouristic,* focusing on the activities or behaviour of the individual, or *psychometric,* focusing on the (measurable) qualities or characteristics of the individual. To replace these traditional views, Svensson (1996) and Sandberg (1994) contended that the concept of competence should be viewed as relational, holistic and contextual. In this framework, competence is not just a set of work tasks to be fulfilled or attributes of the individual to be applied to the tasks, but it is a quality of the relationship between the individual and the actual situation. With regard to the interactive character of professions within health care, this aspect cannot be overemphasised. Approaches to the management of care of individual patients are adapted and changed in interactive processes with sensitivity to matters of specificity and particularity. The care of individual patients is also adapted to change (or lack of change) in the patient's situation, condition and responses.

Rolf et al (1993) argued that professional competence should be viewed as a social praxis or process, where know-how is practised and renewed through the professional's reflection. In emphasising these processes as practical activities (derived from research, education and practice), Rolf et al acknowledged the importance of a practical knowledge tradition.

The influence of context

Every profession has its own frames of understanding, its own tacit rules for how arguments are made and its own traditions for what counts as a valid form of reasoning; these constitute the discourse of the profession (Säljö 1994). As participants in the educational process of their curricula, undergraduates (and other professional entry students) gradually become members of the cultural and discursive community they are about to enter as professionals. The norms for what is regarded as important and relevant are not made up by individual professionals; rather these norms constitute the socially shared and institutionally set framework within the limits of which professionals act out their roles (Mishler 1986). Rolf et al (1993) argued that it is important for students to develop both a practical and a discursive awareness of their profession. Practical awareness implies being knowledgeable about the practical tools available to the profession. Discursive awareness implies being knowledgeable about the traditions, ways of reasoning and unspoken rules of thumb that characterise the profession.

Knowing *in* a profession (the repertoire of theories and techniques) is as important as knowing *about* the profession (the traditions and perspectives of the profession). This knowledge is essential for the further development of the profession. Within this construct is located an awareness of collegiality and the importance of collaboration in sharing and authenticating developing ideas in order to legitimise their place in professional knowledge.

Schön (1983) described the cultural and discursive aspect of professions as differences in the constants brought by various professionals to their reflection-in-action. These constants are: (1) the media, languages and repertoires that practitioners use to describe reality and conduct experiments;

(2) the values and norms they bring to problem-setting, to the evaluation of inquiry and to reflective conversation; (3) the overarching theories by which they make sense of profession-relevant phenomena; and (4) the role frames within which they set their tasks and through which they bound their institutional settings. Schön argued that constancy of appreciative systems is an essential condition for reflection-in-action. It is what makes possible the initial framing of problems. The influence of the communities of practice on the way professionals construct their knowledge is further addressed in Chapter 5.

The reintroduction of technical rationality as the epistemology of practice: a paradox

The changing conditions and the economic cutbacks within the health care sector that the western world has faced during recent years are symptomatic of the drive behind the current emphasis on and call for evidence of effectiveness of health professionals' performance. The professional discourse of many health professions today includes a desire to rise from origins based frequently in craft traditions and strictly experiential knowledge, and to develop into modern, research/evidence-based professions. This has been somewhat achieved by thorough meta-analyses of current research, through evaluations of research results, and of course by conscious design and completion of rigorous original work by researchers. In the best of worlds, these various critiquing activities strengthen the confidence and positioning of the practitioners.

Professions are faced with hard-core challenges to justify their position in the competitive health care community where resources are limited. The search for evidence of treatment results certainly provides answers that, at face value, are irresistible. But this is not sufficient for the future development of the health professions. It is of utmost importance that practitioners are also aware of the need to define and/or recognise criteria that define what counts as evidence. (This is discussed in Chs 6 and 11.) If the objectivist research paradigm and the extreme evidence-based perspective (in which only empirical research knowledge counts as evidence) are given priority as the only bases for professional knowledge, professionals are then themselves reintroducing a technical rationality as the epistemology of practice. Technical rationality as the single epistemology of practice constructs a paradoxical situation for practitioners. On the one hand, practitioners strive for legitimisation of their activity through decontextualised and general research evidence. On the other hand, most health professions are at the same time striving to adopt a more client-centred approach to health care, in which the uniqueness of the single case rather than the generalised, strictly evidence-led approach is emphasised.

THE NEED FOR A RENEWED AND CRITICAL UNDERSTANDING OF REFLECTIVE PRACTICE

A reflective practitioner deliberates on professional practice and on the knowledge base of clinical judgement and reasoning. Inherent in the concept of a profession is the guarantee that assessments and choices for actions are deliberate, well founded and not arbitrary (Juul Jensen 1983). Thus, considering oneself to be a professional practitioner is epistemologically indicative of having understanding, judgement and action within one's sphere, including the evaluation of the outcomes of one's actions (Thornquist 1988).

Research within the health care domain often mirrors an approach characteristic of the medical profession, in which a medical diagnosis is used as the variable against which intervention or treatment is measured. A medical diagnosis is the result of the deliberation and assessment of the medical professions, but this diagnosis often constitutes no more than the starting point for the careful assessment and deliberation of other health care professions. This deliberation and assessment deals with aspects such as problems of function, need for help, need for information. The ongoing assessments, evaluations, adjustments and adaptations that follow and that form important parts of the interactive health care disciplines are neither named nor framed by medical diagnoses per se. On the contrary, all health care professionals know how problems of function and need for information differ between patients sharing the same medical diagnosis. Further, people with quite different diagnoses can share problems such as the need for a specific kind of intervention, or a wheelchair, or exercises enhancing balance, or feeding or indepth information. Obviously the medical diagnosis is not the sole critical factor influencing the choice of interventions in health care. Instead, health care workers' diagnostic processes can be conceived of as an active interpretation enterprise (Thornquist 2001a, 2001b).

It is not enough, however, for practitioners to see that some research fails to address pertinent aspects of professional practice and fails to recognise the role of clinical judgement in practice. It is imperative that research identifies and addresses aspects of practice that practitioners perceive to be pertinent. The practitioner of the 21st century needs to take responsibility for this ongoing articulation of research topics that need to be addressed. Such research will help create and promote a deeper, more relevant understanding and evaluation of practice as well as create and develop the knowledge base of practice.

Practitioners must therefore foster a reflective and also critical stance, striving to uncover premises and presuppositions underlying everyday practice that are not currently reflected in research or articulated in practice knowledge discourse. These premises and ways of thinking ultimately decide how patients' problems are named and framed, both in practice and in research. These (more often than not) unreasoned premises decide how problems are met and treated and how the outcome is evaluated. If the premises underlying practice and research are elucidated, together with a conscious reflection on what is meant by knowledge and evidence, it will be possible to describe more adequately and to evaluate critically professions and their practice. Such descriptions and evaluations may further the development of the skills, knowledge and competence of the professions, testing, refining and strengthening those areas which meet the aims and efforts of the profession, and eliminating those which are seen as not furthering the aims of professional practice. Practitioners therefore need to be challenged to reflect on and articulate the intuitive criteria which underpin professional judgement, to take knowledge which resides in the experiential dimension, test it and expose it to public critique and application.

Bringing the functional relation between focused attention and tacit awareness into reflection-on-practice

In his thesis on tacit knowing, Michael Polanyi (1966) highlighted an important feature of knowing that enhances the possibility of reflection-on-practice. In knowing, we rely on our awareness of some particulars, in order that we can attend to something else. That is, any focused attention relies on a tacit awareness of particulars not attended to at that moment. This is what Polanyi labelled the *functional relation* between the two terms of tacit knowing. He argued that we are aware of the first term only by relying on our awareness of it when attending to the second term. As an example from physiotherapy practice, attending to the gait of a person could be shown to involve reliance on a tacit awareness of a number of particulars, such as the scope and rhythm of separate movements of limbs and joints and the relations between them. This example also shows us the result of having been trained in a particular profession. Physiotherapists have been trained to attend to certain things. The attention focused on such particulars as the movement of separate joints and limbs is subsequently turned into a subsidiary awareness of these particulars in the overall attention to the gait as a whole. Some of these particulars have been spelled out in training, others are such that they are simply acquired in the process of learning and practice. But it is important to foster reflective attention to one's assessments and modifications in practice, identifying particulars and the ways of thinking underlying them. Not all the particulars guiding practice that practitioners learn in the course of their professional education are well founded, and many may not have been subject to deliberate scrutiny or critique. Other (tacit or inherent) features of professional practice may be both well-founded and deliberate, but need to be spelt out in collegial discussion and framed for research.

In practice as a whole, as well as in reflection, practitioners can be said to work within the tension between the confidence needed to support the ability to act and the scepticism inherent in evaluation and critical reflection.

Polanyi's (1966) thesis that any focused attention relies on a tacit awareness of particulars not attended to at that moment implies that when we focus attention on certain particulars that help form clinical judgements we are tacitly relying on other particulars which cannot be critically attended to at that precise moment. This reasoning is also applicable when we are talking about reflection about practice. In reflection about practice or research, a critical and slightly sceptical approach is needed, but this sceptical approach relies on a non-sceptical awareness of matters that are for the moment taken for granted. The functional relation of the terms of tacit knowing shows us that reflection and critical thinking can work only through piecemeal attention and reflection, and that we cannot question or scrutinise all our assumptions at the same time. Background knowledge, such as that shared in a profession, is often trusted, or relied upon without questioning. Reflection on this background knowledge as a prelude for knowledge testing must of necessity be piecemeal, for it would be impossible to challenge all shared professional assumptions at the same time. We can reflect on them selectively, singularly or in small groups, but not collectively at the same time (Kalman 1999). As Popper (1965) stated, at any given moment we take a vast amount of knowledge for granted, but this does not mean that we have to accept any of it as certain or ultimately established.

It is important for the reflective practitioner to acknowledge the nature of this situation, so as to be aware of the ongoing need for reflection on practice. Fruitful reflection and collegial discussion of the basic assumptions inherent in professional practice lead to a common acceptance of a considerable amount of background knowledge. On the other hand, uncritical acceptance of some shared tacit background knowledge and assumptions may also be responsible for some of the difficulties of professionals in reflecting on praxis and articulating its problematics. Those shared background assumptions may themselves give rise to some of the problematics they sought to solve in the first place. Consequently there is a tension between the acceptance of, and reliance on, background professional knowledge for salient and adequate reflection on the circumstances of practice, and the open-minded questioning and critical reflection that do not rely on taking those same things for granted. This is what makes professionals their own both best and worst critics.

The importance of subjecting theoretical concepts to reflection

Some important concepts for conscious reflection are *evidence, knowledge, perspective* and *concept*, and these concepts are themselves important tools for further reflection. A difficult but more important challenge is seeking to understand perspectives and concepts that are perceived to be 'natural' and thus largely unnoticed and unquestioned. Another interesting aspect of this invisible, taken-for-granted world of tacit knowledge underpinning practice and research is the interdependence between experiences, conceptualisation and our linguistic representations. In the philosophy of science this interdependence is known as the theory-ladenness of observations. Popper, writing about observation and interpretation of observations, stated:

My point of view is, briefly, that our ordinary language is full of theories; that observation is always observation in the light of theories; that it is only inductivist prejudice which leads people to think that there could be a phenomenal language, free of theories, and distinguishable from a 'theoretical language' (Popper 1968 [1934], 59, n.*1).

Popper further argued:

Observations, and even more so observation statements and statements of experimental results, are always *interpretations* of the facts observed; ... they are *interpretations in the light of theories* (Popper 1968 [1934], 107, n.*3)

Today the concept of *evidence* has achieved the status of a seemingly self-explanatory and self-justifying concept, to the extent that it is considered so self-evident and natural that it need not enter the domain of practitioner's reflection and deliberate argumentation, rather it 'just needs to be acted upon'. However, deeper scrutiny of the origins of this concept provides a different understanding of its meaning. Historically, the philosophical concept of evidence was intended to mean an immediate insight, as opposed to a discursive insight. Discursive knowledge is reached through intermediaries, through deduction, but not directly or instantly. In discursive thought, thinking is developed step by step, with words added to make a chain of propositions. In contrast, the term *evidence* once denoted 'what we regard as self-evident', that which does not stand in need of explanation. However, with time this view came to be regarded as being problematic; it treated evidence as a psychological state, as a private phenomenon. This view created problems in a world of science which contends that such individual and possibly contradictory perceptions of the self-evident are not necessarily correct. Instead, knowledge is now considered to be something that can be, in principle at least, intersubjectively tested. This basically sceptical perspective is one of the fundaments of the scientific approach today.

It was in Anglo-Saxon philosophy that today's notion of evidence began to be used. That is, when we say that a fact gives supporting evidence, we mean that this fact gives good grounds for believing something to be the case. This understanding is close to the murder trial's understanding of evidence, where, for example, the fingerprint on the gun gives evidence to support a belief about who committed the murder. In this understanding, the concept of evidence is almost synonymous with confirmation, or what Popper would have labelled corroboration. A hypothesis is corroborated when data (e.g. observations, experimental data) that are sought to test the hypothesis are in line with the hypothesis. But it should be remembered that even though data support the hypothesis which is then corroborated, this still does not equate with a guarantee that the hypothesis is true. It is rather a conditional truth, sufficing until further notice (e.g. further research which supports or negates the hypothesis).

In other words, this understanding of evidence fits well with our ordinary everyday understanding of the word, where there are many different kinds of evidence that provide proof or strong probability. We need to remember that what counts as proof or evidence differs between different traditions of science and knowledge, and that at its best there is a 'family likeness' between these concepts of evidence.

Evidence-based knowledge in the health care domain – antithetic to reflection?

The strongly instrumental view of the relationship between science and professional practice, presented in the section on technical rationality above, has been especially dominant within the natural sciences and medical science, but has also had strong representation at times in the social sciences and humanities. The currently stressed concept of evidence came into use within the branch of medical science that has historical roots in pathological anatomy and experimental physiology using controlled trial research and statistics; that concept then spread throughout the health care system (Ekeli 2000a). This view has constituted a narrow, but not necessarily precise or adequate concept of evidence. This is problematic, as Ekeli (2000b) has argued, because randomised clinical trials are put forward as the desired model for attaining evidence. These trials most often take a medical diagnosis as a starting point instead of being framed in the interactive approaches and functional assessments of other health care professions. Randomised controlled studies are considered to be the highest ranked way of obtaining research knowledge in evidence-based medicine. (See Ch. 9 for a detailed analysis.)

The programmatic use today of what is labelled evidence-based knowledge in the health care domain could also be considered antithetic to reflection, because evidence-based medicine is supposed to give guidelines for professional action over and above the person-to-person interaction in the clinic.

It could even be argued that such an attitude towards research is antithetical to the scientific spirit itself. Scientific investigations, their results and the necessary, albeit often missing, reasoning for why the investigations are framed and the results interpreted as they are, are in principle supposed to be able to be put to test or judgement by any person. Juul Jensen (1983) argued that the label 'profession' is supposed to be a guarantee that the assessments and choices for action are deliberate, well-founded and not arbitrary. Thornquist (1988) stressed the point that inherent to the notion of being professional is the requirement to be able to evaluate one's own professional practice, and further that health care professions need to develop a generally critical and analytic stance to reviewing their own practice as well as the practice of the profession as a whole. Reflective practitioners who aim to found professional action on research cannot do this by way of uncritical implementation of guidelines based on research. Instead, practitioners need to deliberate actively on research and practice in general, and specifically to reflect on whether the research in question is pertinent to the practice in question.

Recognising the multifaceted dimensions of reflection

It is quite unlikely that the medical sciences could provide the sole or comprehensive model of scientific approach to knowledge generation for the human as well as the physical sciences across the health care professions. Instead, the careful deliberation and reflection that characterise the practice of health professionals are likely to be better matched by research traditions such as hermeneutics, critical theory, phenomenology, existentialism and structuralism. Not only does the interactive character of the health care disciplines have to be recognised. It is also important that the reflective practitioner be prepared always to pose questions anew, in practice as well as in research, and be prepared to argue about what counts as the correct framing of a problem and what counts as evidence in specific circumstances (see also Chs 6 and 11).

Reflection is in itself a practice, and as such it belongs to an epistemology of practice inherent to these other scientific traditions described in the previous paragraph. An epistemology of practice also stresses the practical nature of seeking and gaining knowledge in our society, and is able to deal with scientific research as one practice among others. This means that an epistemology of practice recognises a variety of ways of achieving knowledge, it does not only rely on knowledge obtained through research according to the rules of natural science.

The difference must be acknowledged between distanced reflection about practice (that may be done after the day's work or while reading research reports) and the reflections, adaptations and responses in situation-specific moments that require instant action. The difference between these two modes of reflection is not that the latter is done without thought, but that our focused attention in situations that require instant action does not allow for the same stepping back from or out of the situation. Still it is possible 'to a certain degree, maintain a reflexive dialogue between the I and the self. The I monitors as it were what the self does while doing it' (van Manen 1995, p. 40). This continued process and use of reflection also echoes what has been shown to be an important part of the ongoing development of expertise in clinicians, where 'expert practice is the result of continual reflection on past and current professional and personal life experiences' (Martin et al 1999, p. 232).

IMPLICATIONS FOR THE EDUCATION OF HEALTH PROFESSIONALS

In the following section we consider some implications of this discussion for education. How can reflective practice be fostered? Can educational strategies such as learning contracts, reflective journals, reflective writing and critical accountability inculcate a commitment to a continued practice of effective self-critique? Do educational devices such as these promote or hamper the development of reflective practitioners?

If undergraduate education programmes are designed to prepare students for a career of work in changing health care contexts then it should be expected that the development of an ability to understand and use processes of reflection will be central to the curricula. One of the key concerns for modern education in health care is to promulgate attitudes and skills that are relevant to working with change: changing practice and changing contexts of care. This highlights the need for students/practitioners to learn how to design and lead change to improve patient care (Leach 2001). It also encompasses the need to learn how to collaborate with new ways of working in multidisciplinary teams, how to work in a variety of care settings and how to comply with an acceptable standard of governance of health care resources, whilst still aspiring to meet professional objectives. The place of reflection in the curriculum for undergraduate education will be governed by the extent of recognition of the epistemological assumptions underpinning practice and the challenge they pose.

Reflection as a means of learning on the individual level as well as the collective level

It can be argued that students fundamentally need a critical awareness of the paradigmatic features of their profession. By paradigmatic features we mean:

- the philosophy of purpose
- the cognitive processes of practice
- the recognised discrete health goals of their specific profession.

Students need to understand what their profession contributes to health compared with other professions. They also need an overview of the origins and history of their profession: influences on its development, critical points of change in methodologies and working contexts, historical features which mark major changes in approaches to or focus of care. Above all they need to understand how the development of their professional practice and the knowledge they generate through practice can add to the development of the profession as a whole.

This sense of not only being consumers of a ready-made amount of knowledge, but also being part of the development of their chosen profession can drive students' motivation to work consciously and thoughtfully in order to develop their professional knowledge. Eraut (1994, p. 12) suggested that much practice knowledge is derived from experiential learning, when new knowledge is generated from the reorganisation, distillation and sharing of personal experience. It follows that the conscious act of reflection becomes an important tool of professional development, a central aspect of the learning process of each student.

According to whether the purpose of reflection is seen as the improvement of immediate practice or as professional development (and the consequent improvement of long-term practice), it can determine whether the practitioner engages in it prior to, during or after a clinical interaction. The simple proposal of the educationalist, Dewey, who wrote extensively about the importance of reflection in learning, acknowledged both the immediate and long-term purpose. He argued for an 'active persistent and careful consideration of any belief or supposed form of knowledge in the light of grounds that support it and the further conclusions to which it tends' (Dewey 1933, p. 9). This suggests a conscious and continual process of awareness of practice underpinned by an assumption of an infinite potential for improved ways of acting. Reflection in learning conveys a sense of a dynamic flow of activities, of changes in appraisal within changing conditions and of a central recognition of the continual flux and change of interactions, requiring continual observation and response.

Importantly, reflection conveys the continuity of change which is intrinsic to an epistemological perspective of knowledge being contextual and unfolding. It is the full understanding of this concept that underpins what the act of reflection tries to capture. This crucial concept is imparted in an education process which encourages collaborative ways of working, which requires students to reveal their reflections and decision-making assessments and which involves students in framing the task and the criteria on which the task is to be judged. Taking a constructivist view of knowledge demands that the notion of the superiority of the teacher to the student as learner is dismantled and replaced with a view of mutual participation in knowledge generation which is relevant to professional practice.

Both Dewey and Schön considered that reflection is most often stimulated by states of doubt or hesitation, but Dewey endorsed the authenticity of a continuous state of questioning practice. The adoption of a principle of fallibilism in professional work can be seen at the heart of contemporary health care. Clouder (2000) pointed out that reflection is not an end in itself but rather a means to an end. It can be seen as an essential component of both clinical reasoning and clinical audit when it is utilised in the reasoning process of intervention and in retrospective reflection on the improvement and development of practice. The student needs to become aware of all the dimensions of reflection and the processes which constitute it. Kember et al (2001) particularly distinguished components of thoughtful action and introspection, believing the latter to be concerned with emotions and attitudes and with a potential for self-doubt which can lead to a clouding of views and progress if not drawn into peer discussion and appraisal.

An implicit and explicit curriculum to support the pivotal importance of the processes of reflection thus aims to foster recognition of the reflective aspects of both immediate clinical decision-making and long-term professional development. The epistemological assumption of the social construction of knowledge strongly supports strategies for the development of reflective abilities which can be demonstrated throughout the curriculum. Key areas of activity which would support the social construction of knowledge in action are a staff–student relationship of collaboration in which both are recognised to be equally engaged in knowledge development; a concept of curriculum which extends seamlessly between classroom and clinic; and the use of assessment methods which put students in charge of the development of their expertise and clinical prowess.

The need for student-centred approaches to education

An open and equal staff–student relationship is critical to foster questioning and prioritising of alternative approaches and methods of practice in a general culture of learning which encourages and authenticates debate, scepticism and enquiry. Shared discussion and peer review which is regarded as the norm in sessions of reflection built into the syllabus can ensure that reflection is seen as central to the process of professional practice and learning in both the academic and the clinical setting. As Eraut (1994) indicated, unless supported and demonstrated by colleagues in the workplace, reflection can be seen as inauthentic behaviour and an intrusion from the world of academia. A concept of a community of practice (Ch. 5) that embraces the classroom and the clinic can do much to facilitate reflection on the lived experience of students which contributes purposefully to the experiential generation of their knowledge. Clinical supervisors and faculty alike need to consider the practicalities of fostering reflection in the curriculum. Time is an issue that must be addressed in this process. The amount of time required for reflection is not yet fully appreciated. In both classroom and clinic settings there are time pressures which can blur the distinction between note-writing and reflective writing, and between reporting and oral reflecting. Such misunderstandings can hinder the development of a relationship between student and teacher or student and clinical supervisor which encourages open and frank discussion of ideas.

Bringing the assessment system into harmony with the notion of reflective practice

Acknowledgement of the epistemological foundations of autonomous reflective practice can be equally demonstrated through an appropriate assessment style which places value upon situational factors of clinical practice and rationales for the practitioner's decisions. Research in higher education has shown that assessment is one of the most powerful forces for influencing student learning. The influence of assessment on approaches to learning is not only exerted by the form of assessment per se; the students' anticipation of the examination and marking also influences how they go about their learning activities (Ramsden 1997). Ramsden summarises the research findings regarding the influence of assessment on students' learning, pointing to some key features: assessments comprising an overwhelming amount of curricular material or utilising inappropriate assessment questions and techniques push the students into surface approaches to learning, which often lead to an incomplete understanding of the subject matter. As Kember et al (2001) suggested, surface learning rather than deep learning is encouraged by assessments which demand only pure recall, by over-formal relationships with staff, by didactic teaching methods which provide little time for interaction and by teaching which fails to capture the interest of the students. A lesson that was learnt from research on student learning in higher education in recent decades is that great efforts are needed to block surface approaches and to enhance deep approaches to learning. To accomplish the enhancement of deep approaches, a greater flexibility and variety in learning tasks and in forms of teaching has been suggested and believed to be beneficial to students in all subject areas (Ramsden 1997).

Recently there have been moves for a structured approach to instigate reflection in an explicit curriculum, with much discussion concerning the format it should take. It could be argued that this strategy appears to be more concerned with processes of audit rather than student ability. Interest has been raised in many professions by the notion of portfolios which can demonstrate a student's progress. Although portfolios and reflective writing can be useful ways to document experience, the quality of reflection within them needs to be assured if they are not to become simply a record of achievements (Stewart & Richardson 2000) rather than evidence of an integrated process of metacognition and introspection. The long-term gains of keeping a portfolio are still to be fully assessed (Smith & Tillema 2001). In both undergraduate courses and clinical practice the increasing use of guidelines and assessment criteria can further bias against the spontaneous use of reflection and of tools to facilitate it. Writing down one's thoughts in a reflective diary, examining the learning process through procedures of evaluating critical incidents, carrying out analyses of individual strengths and weaknesses, opportunities for and threats to development (so-called SWOT analyses) can all assist reflective processes. It is important, however, to realise that concern with assessment outcomes can cloud the essential purpose of reflection for continuing professional development and can emphasise a procedure with the endpoint of an assessment mark rather than a process of practice (Stewart & Richardson 2000, Smith & Tillema 2001). Perhaps the most crucial need is fostering an understanding of reflexivity in students which will bring a critical consciousness of their cognitive activities in reflection.

THE CORE RESPONSIBILITIES OF THE REFLECTIVE PRACTITIONER

In the remainder of this chapter we seek to formulate the core propensities of the reflective practitioner. Health care professionals of the 21st century are educated within curricula largely created and managed by academics, but their respective fields of practice most commonly reside outside the universities. Nevertheless, we should expect university educational programmes to educate students to adopt a critical and reflective stance towards their knowledge and their activities. This means that reflection on practice can result in practice-generated knowledge. It also means that what Boyer (1990) labelled the scholarships of academia become critically transferred to the field of practice, appearing in a different guise that must be recognised by the reflective practitioner. Boyer described four kinds of scholarship that are characteristic of academics and form an interdependent whole of their knowledge base. While these scholarships particularly referred to the professoriate, their exploration has relevance in this chapter because we consider practitioners to be critical and reflective users and generators of knowledge. The term *scholarship* could in this context be seen as the responsibilities of being a professional within academia, which include the *scholarship of discovery, the scholarship of integration, the scholarship of application* and *the scholarship of teaching*.

By the scholarship of discovery, Boyer referred to the involvement and participation in research as essential for discovering new knowledge. The counterpart of the scholarship of discovery could, from the viewpoint of the reflective practitioner, be the responsibility for constant *attentive inquiry*. The reflective practitioner needs to develop a constant attentive and critical stance towards unique situations. Attentive inquiry recognises and records the different modes in which new knowledge emerges; this recognition includes an awareness of the source through which new knowledge is derived. The scholarship of integration means the ability to give meaning and perspective to isolated facts, and to make connections across other disciplines to place the specialities in a larger context through collaboration.

The scholarship of application means, in Boyer's words, application of knowledge in its widest sense. Boyer emphasised that the term *application* itself may be misleading if it is interpreted to mean that knowledge is first 'discovered' and then 'applied'. On the contrary, in agreement with Eraut (1994), Boyer (1990) argued that the terms are interdependent, and that the very act of application itself can lead to a new intellectual understanding. For the reflective practitioner the scholarship of application encompasses the responsibility of applying a *sensitivity for idiosyncrasies*. It does not imply that there should be no general guidelines or collective knowledge within the profession, but rather it points at the practical wisdom applied by practitioners. Practical wisdom includes the wise and critical scrutiny, in relation to the unique circumstances of the single case, of evidence-based recommendations and of the research upon which they were based.

The scholarship of teaching, Boyer (1990) argued, involves not only the transmission of knowledge, but also its transformation and extension through interplay and mutual exchange between teachers and students. For the reflective practitioner, these exchanges could be described as the responsibility to bring about *dialogical learning*. As we have emphasised in this chapter, the need for student-centred education and an equal relationship between teachers and students is paramount in approaches to the education of professionals for the 21st century. It is a learning process on two levels, the individual as well as the collective level. It is a matter of building and developing reflective practice in relation to and in collaboration with newcomers to the profession.

Finally, the scholarship of integration in Boyer's terminology would appear in practice as the responsibility for accomplishing *reflective collaboration* and cooperation across disciplines. It encompasses collegiality in sharing and authenticating developing ideas to legitimise their place in professional knowledge, but also emphasises the need for recognising the specific contribution of the professional.

CONCLUSION

This chapter has reviewed the origins and evolution of the notion and behaviour of *reflective practitioners*. We have presented a new model of the reflective practitioner, redefining the term to address the compelling needs and drives of the 21st century. The responsibilities of attentive inquiry, sensitivity for idiosyncrasies, dialogical learning and reflective collaboration are the hallmarks of reflective practitioners of the 21st century. They should be addressed in the education of health professionals and included among the topics necessary for reflective practitioners to reflect upon.

REFERENCES

Ball, S. (1994). Intellectuals or technicians: the urgent role of theory in educational studies. Annual address to the *Standing Conference for Studies in Education*. London: Royal Society of Arts Examinations.

Boyer, E. L. (1990). *Scholarship Reconsidered: Priorities of the Professoriate*. Lawrenceville, NJ: Princeton University Press.

Clouder, L. (2000). Reflective practice in physiotherapy education: a critical conversation. *Studies in Higher Education*, 25(2), 211–23.

Dewey, J. (1933). *How We Think: A Restatement of the Relation of Reflective Thinking to the Educative Process*. Boston: Heath.

Ecclestone, K. (1996). The reflective practitioner: mantra or model for emancipation? *Studies in the Education of Adults*, 28(2), 146–61.

Ekeli, B. (2000a). Med 'kunnskapsbasert fysioterapi' baklengs inn i fremtiden? *Fysioterapeuten: Tidskrift for Norske Fysioterapeuter*, **67**(10), 21–6.
Ekeli, B. (2000b). Med 'kunnskapsbasert fysioterapi' baklengs inn i fremtiden? Evidence Based Medicine som konserveringsmiddel. *Fysioterapeuten: Tidskrift for Norske Fysioterapeuter*, **67**(12), 17–22.
Eraut, M. (1994). *Developing Professional Knowledge and Competence*. London: Falmer Press.
Juul Jensen, U. (1983). *Sygdomsbegreber i Praksis: Det Kliniske Arbejdes Filosofi og Videnskapsteori*. Copenhagen: Munksgaard.
Kalman, H. (1999). *The Structure of Knowing: Existential Trust as an Epistemological Category*, vol. 145, Acta Universitatis Umensis, Umeå Studies in the Humanities. Doctoral dissertation, Department of Philosophy and Linguistics, Umeå University. Uppsala: Swedish Science Press.
Kember, D., Kam Yuet Wong, F. & Yeung, E. (2001). The nature of reflection. In *Reflective Teaching and Learning in the Health Professions* (D. Kember, ed.) pp. 3–28. Oxford: Blackwell Sciences.
Leach, D. C. (2001). Changing education to improve patient care. *Quality in Health Care*, **10**(suppl. II), 54–8.
Martin, C., Siösteen, A. & Shepard, K. (1999). The professional development of expert physical therapists in four areas of clinical practice. In *Expertise in Physical Therapy Practice* (G. M. Jensen, L. M. Gwyer & K. Shepard, eds) pp. 231–44. Oxford: Butterworth Heinemann.
Mishler, E. G. (1986). *Research Interviewing*. Cambridge, MA: Harvard University Press.
Molander, B. (1993). *Kunskap i Handling [Knowledge in Action]*. Göteborg: Daidalos.
Polanyi, M. (1966). *The Tacit Dimension*. London: Routledge & Kegan Paul.
Popper, K. R. (1965). *Conjectures and Refutations: The Growth of Scientific Knowledge*, 2nd edn. New York: Harper & Row.
Popper, K. R. (1968/1934). *The Logic of Scientific Discovery*, revised edn. London: Hutchinson.
Ramsden, P. (1997). The context of learning in academic departments. In *The Experience of Learning: Implications for Teaching and Studying in Higher Education*, 2nd edn (F. Marton, D. Hounsell & N. Entwistle, eds) pp. 198–216. Edinburgh: Scottish Academic Press.
Rolf, B. (1991). *Profession, Tradition och Tyst Kunskap [Profession, Tradition and Tacit Knowledge]*. Övre Dalkarshyttan: Nya Doxa.
Rolf, B., Ekstedt, E. & Barnett, R. (1993). *Kvalitet och Kunskapsprocess i Högre Utbildning [Quality and Process of Knowledge Within Higher Education]*. Nora: Nya Doxa.
Säljö, R. (1994). Minding action: conceiving of the world versus participating in cultural practices. *Nordisk Pedagogik*, **2**, 71–80.
Sandberg, J. (1994). *Human Competence at Work*. Gothenburg: BAS.
Schön, D. A. (1983). *The Reflective Practitioner. How Professionals Think in Action*. New York: Basic Books.
Schön, D. A. (1987). *Educating the Reflective Practitioner*. San Francisco: Jossey Bass.
Schön, D. A. (1995). The new scholarship requires a new epistemology. *Change*, **27**(6), 26–34.
Smith, K. & Tillema, H. (2001). Long-term influences of portfolios on professional development. *Scandinavian Journal of Educational Research*, **45**(2), 183–203.
Stewart, S. & Richardson, B. (2000). Reflective practice – should it be assessed? *Assessment and Evaluation in Higher Education*, **25**(4) 369–80.
Svensson, L. (1996). *Behovet av ett Relationellt, Holistiskt och Kontextuellt Kompetensbegrepp. [The Need for a Relational, Holistic and Contextual Concept of Competence]*. Unpublished ms. presented at the Department of Education, Göteborgs University, October 25.
Thornquist, E. (1988). *Fagutvikling i Fysioterapi [Professional Development in Physiotherapy]*. Oslo: Gyldendal Norsk Forlag.
Thornquist, E. (2001a). Diagnostics in physiotherapy – processes, patterns and perspectives, part I. *Advances in Physiotherapy*, **3**(4), 140–50.
Thornquist, E. (2001b). Diagnostics in physiotherapy – processes, patterns and perspectives, part II. *Advances in Physiotherapy*, **3**(4), 151–62.
van Manen, M. (1995). On the epistemology of reflective practice. *Teachers and Teaching: Theory and Practice*, **1**(1), 33–50.

3

Revisiting the philosophical roots of practical knowledge

Bernt Gustavsson

INTRODUCTION

This chapter focuses on how, in the last decades, discussion about knowledge has broadened out of a need for us to have a wider understanding of our lives than we have had traditionally. The aim of the chapter is to show the breadth of the concept of knowledge and the diversity of the discussion of knowledge in philosophical debate today. This can help us to understand and reflect on the changing perspectives on what people do in their different activities and professions, including the practical ones. The actual definition of knowledge has for a long time been considered as that generated from a scientific–theoretical understanding. The traditional and standard conception of knowledge is connected with the Platonic definition (400 BC) of *episteme*, from which the word epistemology derives. This standard definition of knowledge as a description of the world's structure and functions states that knowledge emerges from what we believe or hold to be true. What we believe is true must be supported by good arguments, in order for it to be accepted by us as *justified true beliefs*. This axiom is based on the distinction Plato made between personal opinion, which he called *doxa*, and objective knowledge, which he called episteme. The activity we call epistemology is directed towards first, what can make knowledge certain and true and second, what are the sources of knowledge. This perspective of objective knowledge has had a dominant position in our understanding of knowledge in the western world. Traditionally, questions about the origin of knowledge and its foundation are associated with questions of the content of knowledge in different human activities and involve a discussion about the relationship between theoretical and practical knowledge.

This chapter explores the modern debate within the theory of science, showing how it has become accepted that the historical concept of knowledge starts with a view of positivism in which a concept of verified or falsified knowledge is central, and ends with Kuhn (1970) and his concept of paradigm which incorporates a view that connects knowledge to patterns, world pictures and language. In epistemological discussion of different traditions of knowledge, it is feasible to view knowledge as connected to science and research in a multiplicity of perspectives. This means that it is the topic per se, the problem or issue, that decides which perspective of knowledge is most fruitful to adopt in processes of learning or research. The more perspectives we can access, the richer our possibilities of interpretation and our use of a variety of knowledge sources. The demands on control or verification of knowledge are different when applied to knowledge about nature rather than applied to knowledge about humans and society. In short, different forms of knowledge have different characteristics and criteria of truth verification.

This chapter is intended to help contextualise changing views of practice and the legitimacy of practice knowledge over time. First, the central concepts for understanding knowledge and how they have developed historically are described, then the three forms of knowledge as formulated by Aristotle are described in relation to contemporary discussion on perspectives of science and their relevance, examined in a wider reflection on the content and the application of knowledge in practice.

CENTRAL CONCEPTS FOR UNDERSTANDING KNOWLEDGE

During the course of history, the theoretical and scientific understanding of knowledge has been contrasted with two forms of practical knowledge. The Greek concept *episteme* is now accompanied by those of *techne* and *phronesis*. In describing knowledge, Aristotle, building on the works of Plato (400 BC), used three terms. The term *episteme* represents scientific knowledge, theoretical knowledge. *Techne* is used in connection with the knowledge used in the process of production and creativity, denoting the kind of knowledge we need for producing and creating and for manufacturing various products. Handicraft is frequently used as a metaphor and ideal. *Phronesis* represents practical knowledge or wisdom, and is the knowledge used in the processes of social interaction. It is used in connection to an ethically rooted kind of knowledge or understanding of the norms and values through which people work towards their idea of a good life. These three forms of knowledge, the scientific, the practical and the ethical, can be traced back to Aristotle's text *The Nicomachean Ethics* (300 BC), and this view of knowledge has become the starting point for further discussion of the content of knowledge in an increasingly knowledge-dependent society such as ours.

During the 1980s, following technological and economic developments throughout Europe and beyond, the content of practical knowledge and its relation to professional competence became a topic of increasing interest. There has been an important change in the way of looking at how knowledge is actually produced and a growing acceptance that knowledge is created in and connected to the practical activity that humans pursue. Earlier, the expectation was that abstract knowledge was disseminated via experts and added to practical knowledge. Knowledge is now regarded as connected to practical actions and activities. This highlights an understanding of the great difference between routine actions and reflective actions; that is, knowledge is created through the action of reflecting upon existing routines in various activities. Discussion of these issues draws on a number of different philosophical perspectives. One is Ludwig Wittgenstein's view (1921) which distinguishes that which can be said and that which is beyond words. Another is Michael Polanyi's idea (1958) that knowledge rests upon tacit background knowledge, and a third is Gilbert Ryle's distinction (1949) between knowing that and knowing how. The development of society and the need for learning in different sectors of the community have highlighted the description of practical knowledge in relation to different occupations, as a goal for research and for reflection. In particular, the term *reflective practitioner*, coined by Donald Schön (1983), has been used in conjunction with tacit knowledge and knowledge in practice.

The Aristotelian view of human knowledge

The Aristotelian conception of human knowledge focuses on a person's involvement in a number of activities or forms of life. Theory, *theoria*, is the philosophical activity connected to episteme, whereby we reflect on and investigate how existence is realised. The goal is truth and there is an assumption of a world in which we can have knowledge. Theoretical activity thus involves looking at *what cannot be otherwise than it is*. The aim is to formulate general assertions, which include both a description of how something is and an understanding of *why it is as it is*.

A second philosophical activity, called *poiesis*, is connected to techne and involves recognition of what we do when we form, produce and create different products, that is, the means taken to reach a certain endpoint. In this productive activity the goal is to get something out of the activity itself. The activity functions as a means to reach a goal. It may include recognition of craft work, art and poetry, and also reflection on these activities. It is reflection on *what we are doing when we do it*. The activity of poiesis thus acknowledges a link between and draws together elements of theory and practice.

The third philosophical activity characteristic of humans is *praxis*, which is linked to phronesis. Like the other two activities it is practical in character, but it is distinguished from the others in the sense that it describes human relations. It refers to the objective, the very purpose of the action. It has an ethical dimension in that it is to do with social and political values (the word 'ethics' is created from the word *ethos*, our disposition to act in a certain manner, and is regarded as a general theory of action that supports the social art Aristotle called politics). The goal of the activity of praxis thus includes reflection on processes of both episteme (theoretical knowledge) and techne (productive knowledge), in order to understand the full meaning of the good life, or the quality of life of human well-being towards which we strive. It is the integration of episteme and techne in practical wisdom, to know *how to act for the best of human beings*, that is at the heart of phronesis.

These three forms of knowledge are further connected with three forms of rationality or justification, that is, rationality connected with the theoretical, the productive and with meaning. Episteme is made explicit as theoretical–scientific knowledge, techne as practical–productive knowledge and phronesis as practical wisdom based on the meaning of actions. In distinguishing these different concepts of knowledge we can see how our understanding of knowledge has been broadened to encompass not only science and research but also the idea that it is tied to human practical activities and actions. Knowledge is not merely theoretical, it is also practical, it is about *what we know, what we do and how we act*.

Tracing the development of each of these lines of thought in more detail can help to contextualise the task faced by practitioners today in establishing a currency for their practical knowledge.

The historical development of the three forms of knowledge – episteme, techne and phronesis

Episteme develops through history both as epistemology, that is, as a reflection about the nature of knowledge, and also as the scientific form of knowledge. The search for an agreement or correspondence between subject and object is characteristic of science and scientific knowledge, from the work of Descartes in the 1600s onwards. The notion of a mathematical and exact knowledge, Plato's most typical example of episteme, of that which could not be otherwise, was dominant in determining the direction of all knowledge at that time. This line of thinking was preserved and developed in the· Age of Enlightenment through the positivist tradition in which science is regarded to lead progress. The different criteria used for verification and falsification of knowledge have a particular function within scientific theory to maintain a boundary between scientific knowledge and other knowledge. This other kind of knowledge, which is expressed as speculation, values and so on, and termed *doxa* by Aristotle, is termed *metaphysics* in the positivist tradition.

Techne, for Aristotle stood for technique, craft work and art. However, during the Renaissance a process began in which craft work and art became separated from each other. Art became an example of the absence of a strict division between the theoretical and the practical. It could not be tested in the same way as theories and was not immediately useful. However, the artist worked with tools like the craftsman, and ideas had just as much significance as in science. An early example of the difficulty faced in distinguishing the theoretical from the practical was seen in the relationship between mathematics and music. Mathematics was the original image for Plato's episteme, as mentioned above, while music was regarded as a practical activity. In contrast, a second example, proposed by the Italian mathematician Fibonacci (1509), is the *golden section*, or the divine proportion, that is, the series of numbers in which each number is the sum of the two previous numbers. This mathematical proportion, which can be found in nature, for example through the multiplication of species in reproduction, has been of great importance in the development of aesthetics, the set of principles on which good taste and the appreciation of beauty are based. It can be seen that the meaning we associate with the word 'technique' is now significantly narrower than the meaning the Greeks gave to the word *techne*.

Phronesis was regarded by Aristotle as a general virtue, and connected with the process of activities in human relations which was termed praxis. In the Aristotelian understanding of practice there are thus two types of actions: praxis and poiesis. Poiesis is connected with activities of production, while praxis concerns social and political relationships. Both praxis and phronesis came to play a central role in the theology of the Catholic church, but lost significance with secular development. In modern times praxis and phronesis came to be replaced by techne. It has therefore been a recurrent problem to identify praxis as separate from techne. In our time, the general understanding of the practical is how we can be efficient in the means we use to achieve our ends, but recognition of the concept of phronesis declined or partly disappeared until its return with modern development in the 1980s.

Contemporary discussion on scientific perspectives of knowledge

Scientific discussion establishes clear boundaries between different areas. The common and somewhat overused dichotomy between the two cultures of the natural science, the technical and the social science–humanist areas, constitutes not just the foundation for separating academic faculties, but also the different sets of attitudes to knowledge and science. A distinction is further made between different disciplines and between different perspectives of practice within a particular discipline. If we take a neutral view over time, we can observe a generally increased perception of different perspectives on knowledge. The different conceptions of knowledge proposed by philosophers and theoreticians have resulted in a rich number of perspectives of a single activity from which a selection can be made to justify the pursuit of different goals and endpoints. This variety of perspectives can be seen in conflicts about what can be considered as scientific and where the boundaries of knowledge lie.

One of the most frequently discussed perspectives in recent years has been *social constructivism*, in which knowledge is perceived from a sociological perspective, in contrast to perspectives termed 'knowledge realism' or 'essentialism'. For example, the conflict between biologists and sociologists becomes obvious when we consider how researchers within these two disciplines would study knowledge of humankind. Sociologists would express their findings in terms of power relations between people in construction of knowledge, whereas biologists would present knowledge of humankind as nothing other than medical, physiological or biological. Both these examples are based on the same mistake of reducing all knowledge, or the whole truth of humankind and knowledge, to a particular scientific discipline or perspective. To say, as sociology does, that knowledge is 'nothing other than' social constructions is the same mistake as saying that humans are 'nothing other than' their biological make-up.

Scientific reductionism can be found in all sciences. The continual competition between the sciences for hierarchical position is part of the history of science and is somehow accepted as beyond knowledge as power and truth. Throughout the history of science it is possible to identify a hierarchy of sciences, in which a particular science has occupied the highest position, and consequently is assumed to have the greatest truth-value and thus the greatest power when it comes to determining the dominant interpretation of all knowledge. At one time it was theology, at another time philosophy, then physics, and now, perhaps, both sociology and biology.

As an alternative to scientific reductionism, which involves reducing knowledge and the study of humankind to a final level and a single science, it is possible to envisage a many-sided acknowledgement of all the levels by which we try to gain knowledge and understanding about humans and reality. It might seem self-evident that humankind and knowledge can be understood with the help of physics, chemistry and biology, as well as sociology and psychology, and also with linguistics, aesthetics and theology. What is of interest, however, is to look at the relationship between the different disciplines and the forms of knowledge with which they are connected. When we work in cross-disciplinary settings, as in multidisciplinary health teams, or carry out thematic studies such as those of the quality of life, the different disciplines are forced into dialogue with each other, which in itself produces new knowledge in the form of new interpretations.

A dialogue-based view of knowledge presupposes an appreciation that a complex phenomenon can be understood from different perspectives, and thus requires an openness to different interpretations. The decisive point in the relationship between different forms of knowledge is a mutual respect for the different activities involved. Moreover, when we generalise this fundamental view of knowledge, it means that a pluralistic attitude towards knowledge, with its many different perspectives, is regarded as an enrichment. The decision regarding which perspective to adopt is connected with the level at which we work, in which science, for which goal, the kinds of questions posed and the problem to be addressed and solved. The issue of interest is then what hindrances or obstacles exist with the adoption of a particular approach, and what kinds of difficulty are practically connected with that approach.

Questions of the context of science

A major question in the discussion of knowledge today is whether it is context-free or context-bound. However, a whole spectrum of different concepts, each in its particular way, claims that knowledge is beyond the influence of the context in which it arises and is applied. This concerns the three forms of knowledge discussed previously: episteme, techne and phronesis. With respect to episteme, this is the form of knowledge which, from the earliest times up to the present, has been regarded as objective and free-standing. This tradition has been continued in modern natural science and in neopositivism, where the Vienna School of Philosophy historically led with the ambition to build an exact language and science. Moritz Schlick (1925), leader of the Vienna School, held that the essence of knowledge demands that those in search of it travel to a distant peak in order to look at the thing, to have from there an overview of their relation to all other things. Knowledge is here regarded as synonymous with general theory and this can be compared with its diametrical opposite, in which it is asserted that knowledge is tied to its context.

I myself assert that I haven't achieved any greater distance from the social world in which I live. The normal view is that in order to gain knowledge one leaves the cave, departs from the place, climbs the mountain, to form for oneself an objective and universal standpoint, but I think of staying in the cave, the place, at ground level to then interpret the world of meanings we share.

This quotation is from Michael Walzer (1983, p. 14), one of the communitarian spokesmen. Communitarianism stresses a concern for the common and the social, and takes its ideas from the knowledge tradition represented by Aristotle, and later by Hegel in 1807 (Taylor 1975). Aristotle asserted, in opposition to Plato, that both knowledge and norms, the theoretical and the practical, *can* be found in context, that is, in the world in which we live. Therefore, empirical investigation is important. According to this view, the norms and values we embody are thus an inbuilt component of the social collective in which we live. This means that the morals, habits and traditions that exist in a society are themselves the preconditions for what people know, what they do and how they act.

The objectivity and the independent character of scientific knowledge were asserted by the majority of analytical philosophers and theorists of science during the first part of the 1900s. The first to break with this pattern was Ludwig Wittgenstein (1953). In his later writings Wittgenstein regarded language as a toolbox which we use to achieve our goals in everyday life. He proposed that we play different 'language games' connected with what we do and what we say. Different language games accompany different forms of life activities, so that the knowledge we possess is used to reach the goals and meanings for which it is useful and to which we can apply them. Knowledge takes on the character of its use: its application constitutes its meaning, more than simply in the manner in which it is expressed. Knowledge is dependent on language. A further major breakthrough in perspectives of knowledge occurred in the theory of science with the publication of Thomas Kuhn's book, *The Structure of Scientific Revolutions* (1970). Kuhn presented his view that scientific knowledge is dependent upon prevailing paradigms. A paradigm is the lens through which researchers regard the world. It is the same as a world view. Accordingly, we can say that science is contextualised internally, from within science itself. The external factors which influence science, society and culture are not part of this conception. Kuhn's investigation is to a large extent based upon perception: how we are made aware of reality, in the form of totalities, which are in their turn dependent upon the patterns through which we regard their reality.

The debate around practical knowledge

An essential school of thought regarding the understanding of practical knowledge is the one which studies knowledge as connected with activities, contexts and concrete situations, i.e. praxis. In this vein, knowledge is not to be regarded as loosely imposed on individuals and activities, but, rather, intimately involved in the ongoing activity itself. It is, as it is now termed, situated. The emerging emphasis placed upon the full understanding and recognition of practical knowledge can be traced through a broadening view of techne and recognition of dimensions of practice which can and cannot be easily articulated. Practical knowledge has been the focus of a number of perspectives, each with the intention of investigating and attempting to determine what characterises this form of knowledge. The following gives a short presentation of these perspectives and their philosophical background.

Practical knowledge in what we do (techne)

A knowledge tradition in which knowledge is regarded as tied to practice is known as pragmatism, and was founded by Charles Sanders Peirce (1839–1914). According to this theory, the starting point for knowledge is located in our habits and our actions (*pragma*). The basic idea is that we act in our everyday manner or in our practical work according to our habits and routines. It is when we are really surprised and habits are broken that something new takes place. To be surprised involves recognition of something we expect to happen not occurring, which implies that we seek something new. Put differently, when we are doing a practical activity and encounter a problem it demands reflection or theory, which we then apply to resolve the problem and develop the activity. Taking this perspective it can be said that knowledge and knowledge development are closely connected with what we do practically.

However, the distinction between techne and phronesis, as described previously, does not exist here. Pragmatism is an example of how *praxis*, action, is reduced to be techne and instrumental knowledge which is connected with what we do, and follows a goal outside the action itself. Pragmatism's great forefathers, Peirce and John Dewey (1859–1952), were strongly influenced by science, but their concept of truth was different from the common view that implies a correspondence between the statement and the object. Peirce and Dewey believed that the truth of knowledge is revealed in the practical consequences of an action. This basic concept has led to pragmatism becoming a theory of knowledge applied by those who work with the development of knowledge in relation to practical activities.

Practical knowledge as the unsayable

During the last century, the first to develop a set of thoughts to investigate the nature of practical knowledge was Ludwig Wittgenstein. This can be observed in one way in his early work (1921) and in a different way in his later work (1953). In the former, the sentence 'what we cannot speak of we must pass over in silence' has been taken as a starting point for understanding what we call tacit knowledge. A distinction is made between what can and what cannot be said, and they are regarded as two different forms of knowledge. The sayable, or that which can be expressed, also called *knowledge based upon assertion*, is synonymous with the scientific knowledge which is expressed in linguistic statements. The unsayable, or that which cannot be expressed, also known as *tacit knowledge*, is knowledge we are not immediately able to express verbally but which we are able to perceive or show in our actions. There have been numerous interpretations of what constitutes tacit knowledge. The positivist interpretation is that Wittgenstein established a boundary between science and metaphysics, so that he could then identify what is significant, namely, exact science. For many positivists, among them Schlick of the Vienna school, this was interpreted as the need for all knowledge to be translated into verbal assertions if it is to be meaningful. In contrast to this view, a second interpretation of Wittgenstein's thinking is that he really regarded the unsayable as the most significant, that which in the end is shown in the meaning of mysticism. A third interpretation is that the unsayable is what can be perceived, or what we can experience, through our deep understanding of the activity. This means that the knowledge which is shaped from long-term familiarity with an occupation (tacit knowledge) can combine with knowledge produced in research (knowledge based upon assertions) to lead development of knowledge of practical occupations. The two forms of knowledge can also come together in dialogue among researchers, authors, artists and actors at collective seminars. In *Philosophical Investigations* (Wittgenstein 1953) the following declaration was the starting point for the pragmatist interpretation of tacit knowledge as common sense (p. 78):

Compare *knowing* and *saying*
how many feet high Mont Blanc is,
how the word 'game' is used,
how a clarinet sounds.
If you are surprised that one can know something and not be able to say it, you are perhaps thinking of a case like the first. Certainly not of one like the third.

Language is played like a game, dependent upon the activity we are carrying out. To be in a language game is, accordingly, to be in a praxis. To master a task means being capable of using language in order to carry out certain operations. However, it also means being familiar with the experiences which have been built up in the area or activity, and the tacit preconditions determining it.

'Knowing that' and 'knowing how'

If we are to follow the growth of practical knowledge chronologically from these philosophical origins, the next stage in this development is Gilbert Ryle and his book *The Concept of Mind* (1949). Here Ryle introduced the terms *knowing how* and *knowing that*. The first refers to skills, the capacity to carry out certain actions, and the second refers to knowing how things are. Ryle regarded knowledge as rational activity, but these forms of knowledge are based upon different kinds of rationality. A theoretical argument is about logical conclusions, while in a practical connection attention is directed towards the activity itself. Knowledge is then tested by what we do. The understanding of what we do arises in the activity itself and knowledge belongs together with what we do. Therefore, to 'know how' involves both what we can do and what we understand, or our insight when acting. The idea thus accompanies us while the activity is taking place. Here knowledge is both being able to do certain operations, a skill, and being able to present a reasoned argument about what has been done.

Knowledge is expressed when one knows what is being done; consequently it is not just a case of acting according to habits or routines. When we do something with an intention and know what we do, we develop practical knowledge. Ryle, like many others in the postwar period, here marked his disagreement with Descartes and the dualist conception of humankind.

Consciousness and the body cannot be clearly separated, which means that what we do and our reflection upon it cannot be separated. The separation between having and not having knowledge is not between consciousness and body, but between what we do in an exclusively habitual and routine manner and what we steadily reflect upon, leading through modification and improvement to something new. Ryle called these activities 'habitual practice' and 'intelligent practice' respectively. Thus far, we have seen that practical knowledge is described as something we do and understand, as a combination of practice and reflection. Spokesmen for pragmatism and also Ryle share the desire to unite practice with theory. However, both the point of departure and the final point for knowledge are practice: what we do. According to Wittgenstein's perspective, as we have seen, parts of our knowledge cannot be expressed in words. One recurring question is whether tacit knowledge must remain tacit, or if one can gradually give verbal expression to it through reflection. An objection to this division of knowledge into the sayable and unsayable is that it cannot be defended, or is based upon an unnecessary dichotomy.

Tacit knowledge or knowing more than we can tell

From a completely different starting point, all knowledge can be described as tacit. The philosophical source for this description is Michael Polanyi and his book *Personal Knowledge* (1958). Polanyi formulated his view as an alternative to a positivist assertion, of which he was deeply critical, which states that it must be possible to express all knowledge in arguments. One of Polanyi's statements which is often repeated is 'we know more than we can tell' (ibid., p. 27). Recognising a face and cycling are two illustrative examples. In a crowd we can easily identify the face of a person we know, for example one of our own children, but we cannot describe it in an adequate manner. We know what we do when we cycle, but we cannot provide a description. A friend of Polanyi's recounted in a letter from the Sudan, where she was working, that parents in a nomadic tribe had strong misgivings about their children beginning school. The reason was that the children knew exactly how many different individual camels there were in a flock of thousands of animals. The parents were afraid that this kind of knowledge would be lost as their children learned more formal knowledge in school.

The concept of tacit knowledge is in this case different. There is always something that is the focus of our attention, whether it is what we are working upon with our hands, or our attempt to solve a scientific problem. This is called 'focal knowledge'. But when our intention is to interpret and understand what we do, how we use the tools we require, then this constitutes a tacit background knowledge. Knowledge builds upon earlier experiences, on traditions that are passed from generation to generation and in craft occupations between master and apprentice. The interpretations we make are dependent upon the traditions in which we have grown up; we use the habits that have crystallised as a result of these traditions. Accordingly, we can say that tacit knowledge in this respect is the precondition for the result realised in the knowledge process.

A question recurrently discussed is whether tacit knowledge is something which can be expressed or whether it cannot be expressed because that would be impossible. If we imagine a floor covered by a carpet as a picture of what could be expressed verbally, we can see that the whole carpet or the floor cannot be covered or described at the same time, but there is not one piece of the floor which is not covered by the carpet. This should mean that our preconditions for knowledge can be made explicit, but not all at the same time.

The examples of tacit knowledge given by Polanyi not only illustrate the idea that what the eyes witness cannot be translated into words; they also pertain to what we can spontaneously perform. One example is the trained pianist who, without extra thought, finds the keys necessary for the melody. When he once learned to play, each and every movement of his fingers required consciousness and had to be practised. In this example we see how what we have learned through practice or in a gradual manner in a certain field becomes tacit knowledge. A more suitable descriptor for this kind of knowledge is intuitive. When we have learned how to perform an action and the body has, so to speak, assimilated it, we can carry it out without having to think. Drivers cannot sit and think in the abstract where the brakes and the accelerator are positioned; doctors cannot look in a textbook every time they are to make a diagnosis.

Linking modes of knowledge to action

The human, in the opinion of Aristotle, is a social animal, a *zoon politikon*. This implies that we become what we are through the social collective to which we belong. For Aristotle this was the Greek State. The human activities presented above as the starting point for our division of knowledge into *theoria*, *poiesis* and *praxis* can also be seen as three forms of life: *bios theoretikos*, an intellectual life; *bios apolautikos*, the felt life or material use; and *bios politikos*, the life of the citizen. In this division there is a ranking, where the highest life form is the theoretical. The sensual life and material life form is the lowest, shared by all, while participation in a political forum is reserved for a minority.

Many have pointed out how this ranking throughout history has resulted in theoretical knowledge gaining the upper hand in the struggle with practical knowledge. From such a perspective, what has happened in the last decade is noteworthy, namely that practical knowledge has received increased attention and become a goal for research, as well as for conception and theory building. One aspect of this development involves studying practical knowledge without the Aristotelian distinction between techne and phronesis, while another tradition makes this distinction clear. This concept of knowledge, connected with *bios politicos*, has been applied in different occupations and kinds of education, especially those involving care.

Practical wisdom

Phronesis is developed by the hermeneutic tradition of interpretation and understanding. Practical wisdom is a part of the interpretation and is practised primarily in the actual situation. The ethical dimension is integral in the custom and habits of action. We achieve the ethical quite simply through acting in an ethically correct manner, just as we become real house-builders by constructing a real house, or we become courageous by acting in a courageous manner. Ethical knowledge is formulated partly in the making of new interpretations, partly through practice in concrete situations.

According to Aristotle, we can achieve wisdom only by working for the good. The goal of wisdom is to accomplish a good life for people, to increase the human sense of well-being and to experience happiness. Happiness in the Aristotelian perspective makes it possible for people to realise their potential and develop their latent capabilities.

Consequently, the question arises as to how knowledge and ethics are connected. In the western world we are accustomed to separating assertions of fact and value. In the modern world, knowledge comes first and ethics, or the sense of value placed upon it, comes second, as a regulative correction of what is perceived to be against the so-called humane or permissible. In the Aristotelian tradition, the ethical is already intrinsic in what we do, in our habits, morals and the ways we are. The norms and the world we inhabit cannot be separated from what we do or the actions we carry out.

Martha C. Nussbaum (1997) is a thinker who has found a way of saying what practical wisdom involves and what can be characterised as important in phronesis as knowledge. The starting point is the local social environment to which we belong. But the norms and the world in which we grow up cannot automatically be taken as given conventions. The new and revolutionary, as suggested by Plato (400 BC), necessitates critical reflection. Nussbaum (1997) supports a view that a life without reflection is not worth living. By critically reflecting on our local community we increase our ability to meet the foreign, the strange. With a critical perspective we move beyond our own perspective; we are able to meet other cultures and horizons of interpretation.

Ethics, Nussbaum (1997) asserts, cannot be reduced to a number of obligations, feelings of bad conscience and what people should do in abstract imagined situations. Ethics involves a broader sphere and deals with life's form and texture as a whole, as it has expanded through the ages. The alternative becomes *eudaimonia*, human well-being, a good and valuable life, as the goal of ethics. Ethical education, therefore, becomes something other than letting yourself be useful, or following a set of rules and norms. To make the difficult decisions in life, or to give form to one's life, cannot be reduced to the rational maximisation of utility. Such choices reflect the whole of humankind, rationality, passions, desire, all our spiritual abilities and the complexity of human life. Practical wisdom, or phronesis, thus consists of the ability to meet concrete situations with sensitivity and imagination. This knowledge incorporates a clear conception of the concrete and complex details that are part of the situation. To make a wise assessment, a process of decision-making is required in order to achieve a resolution of the best actions to take in relation to the concrete situation at hand. The practical circumstances and the situation will thus decide which choices and decisions to make. Nussbaum (1997) compares such deliberations to improvisations in music and drama, suggesting that what counts is flexibility, sensitivity and an openness to the world.

Narrative knowledge

Providing narratives is central to our understanding of our position in time, of knowing where we find ourselves in the history of which we are a part. In our personal history, our interpretation of the present is a product of the past. What we have earlier experienced constitutes a part of our horizon, a limitation in our way of seeing. But at the same time, the interpretation we make at a certain point in time apprehends the future. Our life is interwoven along the three dimensions of time we call the present, the past and the future. We retell stories of what we have been through, but the narrative is told differently at different points in time; it changes with our changing interpretations. The narrative provides us with a way of imagining what has taken place.

If we adopt this perspective on humankind collectively, to grasp what happens with respect to social and cultural development, there are consequences for our relationship to knowledge. There are also consequences for how we regard the relationship between explanation and understanding, that is, between natural science and human science. The person who has developed this line of thought the furthest is the French philosopher Paul Ricoeur. The whole of his philosophical project (Ricoeur 1985) is based upon seeking a bridge which provides a connection between natural science and the phenomenological tradition of understanding the nature of human experience. The narrative links people together with time. Life cannot be grasped without narrative and the human being is defined as a *being who tells stories*. Life as a biological event is a raw material that is interpreted through narratives; through them we leave our lonely existence and become social beings. When we create narratives we unite fact with fantasy. The element of fiction which exists in all knowledge at the same time opens the path which enables us to think beyond the factual to the possible.

SUMMARISING THE CONTEMPORARY DEBATE ON PRACTICAL KNOWLEDGE

In this chapter, discussion of the relationship between the forms of knowledge provides a starting point for discussions of practical knowledge. They are, naturally, in no way mutually exclusive and there is no watertight difference between them. We can regard them as three spheres in which knowledge is discussed in different ways, but by bringing them together we can broaden our perspective on the meaning of knowledge and how we can apply this knowledge to the goals and practical problems we face.

At the same time, it is important to remember that there are limits to the different forms of knowledge, limits which entail risks if transgressed. A latter-day criticism of supporters of practical knowledge has been that practice in modern times has been distorted, becoming the application of technical control over humankind and existence, which is reduced to mechanical problem-solving. And yet, the criteria for objectivity and value-freedom in knowledge as episteme can be developed to include both explanation and understanding. Meanwhile it is equally important to keep in mind that phronesis, as practical wisdom, should never be made into a scientific theory with an objective terminology. The precision and the demands for proof that exist in science can rather be replaced by adequacy and a permanent openness to criticism. What may be wrong in a failure to act adequately may be the perceived social or cultural context in which the practical wisdom was conceived and practised.

A need remains to develop a way of generating activities and education which is capable of creating a good balance between the three forms of knowledge discussed. This requires knowledgeable, insightful and wise people in all groups of society and in all activities. With regard to actions and appropriate means to reach goals, there is no firm ground as a basis for unambiguous decisions, no more than is the case when dealing with matters of health. From this standpoint it can be reasoned generally that the lack of exactness provides an even more valid need for discussion about particular cases. Satisfactory management of individual life events is mastered neither by some special technique nor by any guiding principles; rather, the actors, the persons involved, must themselves seek to determine what is suitable at any moment, and this is the case whether within the arts of medicine or navigation.

REFERENCES

Kuhn, T. (1970). *The Structure of Scientific Revolutions*, 2nd edn. Chicago: University of Chicago Press.
Nussbaum, M. C. (1997). *Cultivating Humanity: A Classical Defense of Reform in Liberal Education.* Cambridge, MA: Harvard University Press.

Polanyi, M. (1958). *Personal Knowledge: Towards a Post-Critical Philosophy.* London: Routledge and Kegan Paul.

Ricoeur, P. (1985). *Time and Narrative.* Chicago: University of Chicago Press.

Ryle, G. (1949). *The Concept of Mind.* Harmondsworth: Penguin Books.

Schlick, M. (1925/1979). *Allgemeine Erkenntnislehre.* Frankfurt: Suhurkamp.

Schön, D. (1983). *The Reflective Practitioner: How Professionals Think in Action.* London: Temple Smith.

Taylor, C. (1975). *Hegel.* Cambridge: Cambridge University Press.

Walzer, M. (1983). *Spheres of Justice: A Defense of Pluralism and Equality.* New York: Basic Books.

Wittgenstein, L. (1921/1963). *Tractatus-Logico-Philosophicus.* Frankfurt: Suhurkamp.

Wittgenstein, L. (1953/1997). *Philosphical Investigations,* 2nd edn, transl. G. E. Anscombe. Oxford: Blackwell.

4

Practice knowledge – its nature, sources and contexts

Joy Higgs, Lee Andresen and Della Fish

INTRODUCTION

Health care professionals working in clinical or fieldwork settings are responsible for the provision of care/services to their patients or clients, ensuring the quality of this care/service, teaching their fellow professionals and contributing to the development of their profession's knowledge base. To achieve these goals, professionals first need to understand the context of their practice. They need to become able to combine knowledge, reasoning and skills in practice, make explicit their practice knowledge, critically appraise their knowledge use and develop their practice knowledge. Finally, they need to use skills of reflection, theorisation and research to critique, refine and generate practice knowledge which can contribute to the public knowledge available for use by their profession. Educators and researchers in the health sciences share these same responsibilities, in order to be able to assist the enhancement of practice through their respective teaching and research roles.

A PRACTICE KNOWLEDGE POSITION

We adopt the following position throughout this chapter:

- We reject the *theory–practice dichotomy* (or separation) as false and misleading, since theory and practice coexist and combine in practice settings; they are interconnected and interdependent, so that whenever one is mentioned the other is also inseparably present.

- In this chapter we are dealing with the intertwined entities of *practice and theory/knowledge* from the immediate practice-setting viewpoint of practitioners and from the more distant viewpoint of academia with its research and education functions. In health-related workplaces, the use and creation of knowledge and the activities of practice are inextricable, and the processes of clinical reasoning and professional decision-making provide the medium for combining all of these elements (Fig. 4.1). In academia we may teach reasoning, knowledge, theory and technical skills, but unless these are grounded in practice they are merely mental gymnastics, academic curiosities or physical prowess. They need the reality and experience of practice to give them significance and meaning. Similarly, research, in the context of the health professions, being the generation of theoretical knowledge, can occur in practice, or can be about or for practice. Theories emerge from practice or are created to explain, explore or extend practice. We recognise that within the development of knowledge, practice is what comes first, and theory is developed from it. This idea is traditionally referred to as 'the primacy of practice'.

In Figure 4.1 we illustrate the relationship we perceive between the core elements of practice and knowledge. Practice as central is represented by the circle which encompasses the various activities and experiences of professional practice. Two intertwining loops (practice knowledge and reasoning)

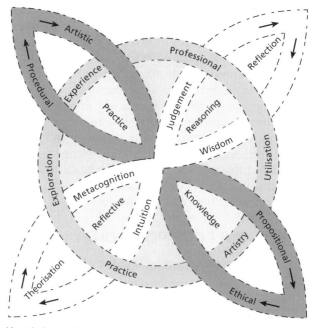

Figure 4.1 Knowledge and practice

are enmeshed in practice. In addition, these processes extend outside the current practice action, representing knowledge and practice development activities (learning, research, theorisation and reflection) which arise from and feed back into practice. The whole diagram has fuzzy uncertain edges and interweaving forms, representing the interactivity between elements and their uncertainty and evolution.

• Understanding the nature of knowledge involves adopting a position about how knowledge is created and recognising that we need a sense of wonderment and curiosity to seek out what we do not know, indeed to recognise that we are ignorant and unaware of many things. In the midst of our changing world practitioners are unaware of much of what we do and why we do it in practice. Knowledge, we argue, is dynamic, context-bound and constructed from different ways of knowing.

• Practice knowledge operates within a number of contexts, including that of the individual practitioner, the practitioner's discipline, the culture, the society and the historical era. These contexts are not separate, but interconnected and interdependent.

ACKNOWLEDGING THE PRACTICE KNOWLEDGE CONTEXT

The nature of practice

Practice in the health sciences is a challenging responsibility that requires health professionals to work in complex situations armed with a rich array of knowledge and practice skills reaching far beyond precise or prescribed knowledge and competencies (which are at times implied through professional sets of competencies or limited views of what constitutes evidence as the basis for practice). Given the often indeterminate nature and settings of practice and the expectations of accountability facing health practitioners as responsible professionals, it is insufficient to view practice as a series of well-defined instrumental problems that can be addressed using one of a number of predetermined solutions. Such fixed solutions would limit the role of the health practitioner to that of an applied scientist whose practice is constrained by application of available research knowledge to identified problems (Schein 1973). In other words, this would mean recognising the 'primacy of theory' as the rationale for how professional practitioners work, which argues that theory comes first and is applied on practice. On the contrary: this chapter is arguing for the 'primacy of practice'.

The traditional view of professional practice, in which theory is thought to be applied to practice in a technical–rational way, is being challenged by a vision of practice in which professional artistry is required to address the uncertainty of practice demands (Schön 1983). Practice and the practice environment are portrayed by Eraut (1994, p. 17) as complex and unpredictable, requiring 'wise judgement under conditions of considerable uncertainty'. Professional practice is an inexact science (Kennedy 1987) or, better still, a blend of art, science, craft and humanity (Higgs et al 2001). This view of practice presents a vision of practice knowledge in which empirical, critical, practical and aesthetic ways of knowing are needed, along with different ways of seeing knowledge, truth and proof, which include but also go beyond 'hard science'. It is our belief that effective professional practice requires creating new understandings during practice. A moral and ethical approach to practice is needed, working in collaboration with clients, employing ongoing critical examination of beliefs and positions, living with a heightened awareness of the potential for errors, and engaging in critical self-monitoring.

The primacy of practice

In his seminal 1949 book on the philosophy of mind, *The Concept of Mind*, Gilbert Ryle called our attention to the arguments for the primacy of practice. He wrote:

Efficient practice precedes the theory of it; methodologies presuppose the application of methods, of the critical investigation of which they are the products ... It is therefore possible for people intelligently to perform some sorts of operations when they are not yet able to consider any propositions enjoining how they should be performed. Some intelligent performances are not controlled by any interior acknowledgments of the principles applied to them (p. 31).

In arguing that some practice actions have no underlying (acknowledged) principles Ryle prompts us to question which of our actions are or are not supported by theory. To answer this question we need to recognise two very significant aspects of professional knowledge. First, since theoretical knowledge is an attempt to explain practice it cannot fully represent the entirety, the essence, the subtleties and the complexities of practice. It is frequently incomplete and inexact, building on what the knower knows, what is currently known (in the field) and what can be known. For example, greater access to the internet places extensive knowledge sources (needing to be critiqued and distinguished from e-junk) at our fingertips and experience in different modes of knowledge generation opens new avenues for practitioners to create further explanations for practice. Second, knowledge is constantly changing, as are the instruments and ways of knowing. Therefore, what we cannot know now as individuals (e.g. due to the limitations of our learning and understanding) may change with the growth of our professional development. And, what the field does or cannot know now (e.g. due to the limitations in our research methodologies or measurement instruments) may be more knowable in the future with advances in technology and shifts in approaches to knowledge generation.

Ryle argued against the myth of the mind as a 'ghost in the machine' of the body. This was an idea bequeathed by Descartes to the 20th century and perpetuated in many metaphors of the mind we employ even today. Ryle contended that we should not imagine that behind intelligent action is the ghost of intelligent thought. Instead, he argued, 'when I do something intelligently, i.e. thinking what I am doing, I am doing one thing and not two. My performance has a special procedure or manner, not special antecedents' (Ryle 1949, p. 32). Fish and Coles (1998) illustrated this idea of knowledge and practice being indivisible, by using the metaphor of the *iceberg of professional practice*. They argue that roughly one-tenth of practice is the visible performance (action), beneath which (invisibly) lie the theoretical knowledge, the beliefs, assumptions, emotions and values which drive practice; these, of course, imbue the whole of the practice iceberg, including the visible part.

When we speak of acting in professional practice involving knowledge, thinking and practice working together, we are commonly referring to overt actions. Thinking can also be considered to be a form of action. If we distinguish between thinking and other kinds of 'doing' then we can recognise that Ryle's proposition of a simple alternative between two positions (the primacy of practice or of theory) is part of a larger complex picture. We would contend that the principal argument inherent in notions of practice primacy is that practice provides the context (goal, purpose, raison d'être) of practice actions, including the action of thinking as well as other more observable actions.

Sociocultural and language perspectives

We have described above the importance of the context and nature of knowledge in understanding the nature of practice knowledge. In this section we explore two key elements of this topic: language and sociocultural contexts.

Language

Language is 'the technique of accessing and verbally reproducing intrapsychic contents' (Torey 1999, p. 83; where 'intrapsychic' means roughly *mental* or *within a particular mind*). According to this contemporary view of consciousness and the mind–brain relationship, the development of language in human prehistory has meant that people have developed the capacity to control percepts directly (what we think, the pictures the brain conjures up), thus accessing and managing our brain's contents. This language capacity provides us with what we know as our own 'self-experience' or self-awareness. This, more than any other single capacity, is what critically distinguishes humanity from all other animal forms. It is the key to our very humanity, and it enables us to learn and to control our environment. Despite this, language is merely a delivery system. Words are never the same as the things they represent.

Language and thought are inextricably causally linked. Hence the history of human knowledge begins with and is coextensive with the history of human language development. We refer here to language in general, not any specific language form, since all known languages are formed in a similar manner out of analogous primary and secondary syntactic structures. Different languages thus vary in detail (vocabulary, grammatical rules) but not in essence.

Culture, language and values

The philosopher Ludwig Wittgenstein (1953) taught that to speak a (particular) language is to inhabit a 'way of being'. Whereas to speak any language at all is to 'be a human being' (as distinct from any other animal form), to speak (and think in) a *particular* language is to be a *particular kind of human being*. It is to inhabit a particular way of being a human. Each of us is uniquely determined by the special qualities of our own language(s), enabling us to enjoy a very different experience of life from those who speak and think in any other tongue.

Far more than being just a tool for communication, language both shapes and limits the way we construct our social realities. It is one of the principal criteria we use for defining a culture. Other criteria include laws, customs, moral codes, religious beliefs and so on, but as none of these are understandable or capable of functioning except through language, and their special resonances exist because of language, language would appear to be the critical determinant of cultural distinctiveness.

The idea of 'culture' is a comparatively recent one, and the historical origins of the term are instructive. The 18th-century thinker Giambattisto Vico of Bologna (1668–1744) is generally credited with being the father both of the modern concept of culture and of the idea of cultural pluralism. Each authentic culture, he taught, has its unique vision and its scale of values. (This does not, however, mean that different cultures are insulated from influence by other cultures.) As they evolve and develop over time, one vision and set of values may be (partially, but never wholly) replaced by another. Earlier value systems generally remain *at least partially* intelligible to succeeding generations. This is the very basic premise underlying virtually all attempts at doing 'history'.

These ideas are crucially important in the history of knowledge. Pre-Enlightenment thinking was dominated by some rigidly held beliefs, for instance, that there exists an ahistorical and eternal 'natural law'. There was a timeless authority that must be obeyed, and any truth possible to be known could have been discovered by anyone at any time. From the contrary viewpoint of cultural evolution and relativity, however, historical (and knowledge) development can be represented by a succession of cultures, each stemming from its predecessor and standing on the shoulders of whatever came before (Berlin 1990).

Subcultures, societies and socialisation

The social dimensions of language and knowledge are ultimately a dense, complex web, full discussion of which would be impossible in a few lines. However, a few principles can be stated, to help students and researchers find their way through the maze of interlocking issues.

The related terms 'social', 'societal', 'society' and 'socialisation' form a family substantially distinct from the notions 'culture' and 'cultural'. These constructs are related, but the two families shouldn't be confused or conflated. The 'social' family of terms refers to everything that emerges at the *interpersonal level, the group and subgroup level, and the intergroup level* within the overall structure and certainties provided by the language, values, customs and 'centre of gravity' of the given language-culture within which the social groups in question operate. The range of matters here is enormous and varied. It includes religious and political beliefs, affiliations and perspectives, gender and social class differences involving speech, values and outlook, as well as local geographical or tribal characteristics involving dialect, manners and style.

It is in this context that we encounter what are popularly called subcultures, such as the subculture that comprises a given professional group (or even subgroups within a larger profession). These professional groups meet together, possibly work alongside one another or in communication, developing a fine-grained subcultural identity. But they exist only for as long as the social bonds are sustained. This is a very different thing from the stronger, historical notion of culture proposed by Vico and the later German philosopher Herder. Culture, in their terms, is a more or less permanent part of individual identity, remaining with you wherever you may travel, whatever occupations or involvements you may enter into, and centrally organised around the language in which you think and speak.

Notwithstanding this underlying cultural foundation, different social subcultures will develop argots, or distinctive ways of speaking and thinking. The professions exhibit a particularly powerful instance of subcultural structuration. It is a commonplace observation that people within a specific profession (x) will naturally tend to think like an x, see the world through the eyes of an x, notice the things an x notices, and ask the questions an x asks about those things. In education and professional development a central focus is learning to think/speak/write like an x. Those outside that particular socioprofessional group, untrained in the disciplines of thought on which the group is founded, would be blind to these insider insights and more or less excluded from the central processes of knowledge formation within that professional practice. It is this capacity to perceive in a special way, then ask particular questions about what one perceives, rather than the possession of propositional knowledge, that critically distinguishes insiders from outsiders in any profession.

Subgroups, professional subcultures, genders and other social affiliations, however strong, do not ever exist in isolation. Persons from other groups can and do enter (at least partially, but often very substantially) into the ways of thinking and the inner experience of being in another group. As with cultural empathy, this process of entering another profession takes more than mere knowledge of the other group. It often takes a considerable act of imaginative insight. But it is possible, because at depth we share a common humanity, arising from our unique brains that have the capacity to reflect in self-awareness upon their own thinking, and, through language, to have meaningful and unambiguous transactions with other minds. This is the ground of our unique human capacity for knowledge.

The historical context

Professions can be classed as *human practices*. The term 'human practice' is an important one, referring to considerably more than merely the things that people do (MacIntyre 1985). For example, manipulating joints is not a human practice but physiotherapy is. A practice, in this rather strict sense, is an organised, cooperative and coherent human activity, generally of a complex rather than a simple kind. The most important characteristic for our purposes is that a human practice needs reference to *why* and *how* it is done. A human practice exists to gain benefits which are obtainable only by doing that particular thing. And a human practice carries within it standards of excellence by which it may be judged. The benefits, as well as the standards, together comprise an integral, inseparable part of what it means to be doing that practice.

By participating in practices (as here defined; for instance, the practices that make up the health sciences) practitioners systematically extend their conceptions of the best uses and modes of practice and extend their power to achieve excellence in the practice. Under this description the things we call 'professional practices' appear as an important *subset* of the entire field of human practices. The professions comprise those particular practices that are formally organised, that regulate entry and membership, prescribe and control the training required for entry and upgrading, are engaged in for remuneration according to schedules of fees, and are committed to particular ethical codes.

The evolution of professional knowledge involves creating knowledge in practice. It is the outcome of reflection by individuals and professional groups on their knowledge and practice. Such professional knowledge is located within the wider history of ideas and the broader knowledge of society. Understanding human practices requires both an appreciation of their philosophical aspects (as above) and of the contribution of history to their development. We need historical knowledge of the nature of any professional practice if we are to recognise its imperatives, constraints and possibilities. Knowledge which has evolved within a practice includes both the history of the ideas contained in the practice, and the history of how people have shaped those ideas and shaped the practice. With this knowledge we can better contextualise our understanding of contemporary professional practice and more effectively work on developing it.

History is much more than an academic discipline. It is our principal repository of credible knowledge about what it means to be human, and about what humans are capable of thinking, doing and being. Our knowledge of the world of people is grounded in our past history, it forms our current history and it lays the foundations for our future history. Two key premises enable us to appreciate the role of history in knowledge generation.

The first notion is the 'history of ideas' (popularised by Isaiah Berlin 1980), which refers to the birth, impact and decline of *ideas* on the human scene. Each profession has its particular history of characters, events and discoveries, but the history of ideas is larger than the history of any particular practice.

The history of ideas deals with the events surrounding the appearance of particular ideas (concepts, notions, ways of talking about things) on the human scene. It seeks answers to the question of 'why things are as they are'. Even within one culture and one language tradition, the fact that we talk about certain things today does not mean our forebears also talked about them, or (if they did) that they meant the same thing by them. The appearance of new and influential ideas at quite specific times and places is crucially important in following the history of human knowledge itself. The ideas (concepts, terms, notions) that people have available to them at a particular time and place profoundly limit what it is possible for those people to think, and consequently to speak and to write. Hence the available pool of ideas at any historical moment will critically determine the extent and direction of possible new knowledge growth, as well as the ways in which existing knowledge is grasped and expressed.

The second notion which underpins the writing and interpretation of history is *historicism*. Historicism refers to 'the recognition that all social and cultural phenomena are historically determined, and therefore have to be understood in terms of their own age … each [phenomenon] has its location in space and time; such phenomena therefore cannot be subsumed under laws of generalisations that transcend the limits of their age or their society' (Stanford 1998, p. 155). Vico, together with Herder, are the founding fathers of modern historicism (Berlin 1980). They denied the possibility of ever establishing final truth in all the provinces of human thought by the application of the laws of the natural sciences.

We have already argued that the evolution of professional knowledge involves creating knowledge in practice, and reflection by individuals and professions on their knowledge and practice. Now we can perhaps see that this professional knowledge needs always to be interpreted within the wider history of ideas and the broader knowledge of society and the evolution of human cultures.

CATEGORIES OF PRACTICE KNOWLEDGE

Professional practice is sound to the extent that it draws richly and critically on a diversity of knowledge sources. Some of this knowledge is tacit. Practitioners possess often wordless understandings arising out of their cultures and communities. They also need knowledge of the physical and social worlds, knowledge of science and technology and knowledge of their own professional culture with its many hues (e.g. ethics, standards and dilemmas) and expectations (e.g. professionalism and accountability).

Ways of categorising knowledge

In western philosophy, knowledge has been commonly thought of in two ways: as propositional knowledge (or 'knowing that') and as non-propositional knowledge (or 'knowing how') (Ryle 1949, Polanyi 1962). Propositional knowledge is derived formally through research and scholarship and includes scientific knowledge (from the sciences), logic (from philosophy) and aesthetics (from the arts). In its most generalised, systematised, organised, publicised and criticised form such knowledge represents the knowledge of the field. Non-propositional knowledge is derived primarily through practice experience. In professional discourse a perceptible hierarchical relationship has developed between propositional and non-propositional knowledge, with the former accorded a higher status. This is particularly evident in the health sciences where knowledge from the biomedical sciences frequently has precedence in determining what counts as evidence. Barnett (1990), for instance, argued that modern society is unreasonably dominated by the cognitive framework of science, to the extent that other forms of knowledge are downgraded and not even regarded as real knowledge. We concur with Barnett's argument that, in a world where problems are not discrete nor solutions definite, we need knowledge beyond science.

One of the most respected post-Enlightenment categorisations of knowledge that still carries currency is that of Vico (Berlin 1980). Vico identified the following:

- *Deductive knowledge* takes certain propositions or assumptions as a starting point and follows where those assumptions logically lead. Vico referred to this knowledge as things that are true either by definition or by deduction from other things which are themselves true purely by definition.
- *Scientific knowledge* requires objectively valid, reliable and reproducible evidence. Only evidence gained by the senses, through observation, description and measurement, may be counted. Knowledge remains 'true' only for as long as it is not objectively refuted; when it fails the crucial test it becomes obsolete, to be replaced by a superior formula/findings.

- *Experiential knowledge* is gained by personal experience. Some crucially important human knowledge exists which is distinct from and not reducible to either scientific or deductive knowledge.

Vico's insights are echoed by Habermas (1972), whose knowledge framework comprises three knowledge interests: technical, practical and emancipatory. We meet similar ideas in the work of Reason and Heron (1986), whose knowledge categorisation comprises experiential knowledge (gained through direct encounter with persons, places or things), practical knowledge (gained through activity and related to skills or competencies) and propositional knowledge (knowledge of things, gained through conversation, reading, etc.).

Ryle (1949) contended that propositional (theoretical) knowledge and procedural (practical) knowledge are the two main divisions of knowledge. He argued that procedural knowledge has primacy; that propositional knowledge *initially* follows rather than drives procedural knowledge. He pointed out that some theory is inside (part of) practice, while other theory is utilised *in* (rather than *applied to*) practice. Ryle asserted: 'intelligent practice is not a step-child of theory. On the contrary, theorizing is one practice amongst others and is itself intelligently or stupidly conducted' (p. 27). Further, 'we learn *how* by practice, schooled indeed by criticism and example, but often quite unaided by any lessons in the theory' (p. 41).

Higgs and Titchen (1995) explored professional knowledge. Their system includes three categories: propositional knowledge, and two forms of non-propositional knowledge, professional craft knowledge (arising from professional experience) and personal knowledge (arising from personal experience). *Propositional knowledge*, derived through research and/or scholarship, is formal, explicit and exists in the public domain. It may be expressed in propositional statements that describe relationships between concepts or cause–effect relationships, thus permitting claims about generalisability. Or it may be presented in descriptive terms which allow for transferability of use. This will depend on how the knowledge has been generated. *Professional craft knowledge* can be tacit and is embedded in practice; it comprises both general professional knowledge gained from health professionals' practice experience and also specific knowledge about a particular client in a particular situation. *Personal knowledge* includes the collective knowledge held by the community and culture in which the individual lives, and the unique knowledge gained from the individual's life experience. According to Carper (1978, p. 20), personal knowledge 'promotes wholeness and integrity in the personal encounter, the achievement of engagement rather than detachment' and requires 'knowing, encountering and actualizing … the concrete, individual self' (ibid., p. 18). This kind of knowing demands of the clinician the involvement or *engagement* of the whole person; his or her thinking, sensing and perceiving. It is the outcome of both personal and professional experiences and crises, accompanied by reflection. Higgs and Titchen (1995) argued that the importance of personal knowledge in professional practice should not be underestimated. This knowledge, including the individual's frame of reference, values and ethical knowledge, influences the individual's behaviour and acts as a yardstick for self-critique in interpersonal interactions.

Personal knowledge, an important idea in the work of Polanyi (1962), is a recurring theme through all these categorisation systems. Eraut (2000, p. 114) refers to personal knowledge (a person's 'knowledge base') as 'the cognitive resource which a person brings to a situation that enables them to think and perform ... this incorporates codified (i.e. public or propositional) knowledge in its personalised form, together with procedural knowledge and process knowledge, experiential knowledge and impressions in episodic memory ... personal knowledge may be either explicit or tacit'.

It should be noted that knowledge in any one category can be (and often is) translated into or subsumed within another category. For instance, knowledge derived from experience can subsequently be transformed into formal, publicly assessable propositional knowledge through theorisation. Propositional knowledge (of the field) can on the other hand also arise through basic or applied research. It can then be extended and particularised through practice experience to become part of the experience of the individual.

In Figure 4.2 we endeavour to capture the various ideas within these knowledge categorisations into a model of practice knowledge. This model includes:

1. propositional knowledge (which describes and predicts)
2. procedural knowledge (which enables action)
3. theoretical knowledge (which explains and interprets)
4. emancipatory knowledge (which empowers people).

The model also:

5. recognises that these types of knowledge overlap, inform each other and can be transformed or extended one to the other
6. acknowledges different ways of generating knowledge through deduction, theorisation, research and reflection on experience.

Knowledge and theory

We believe that practice is theory-based, but not driven by theory (neither personal nor formal theory). In presenting this argument we are introducing a typology of theories comprising first, personal theories (frameworks of

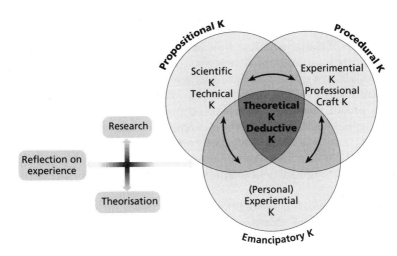

Figure 4.2   Forms of knowledge (K)

understanding or explanatory theoretical arguments created by individuals to make sense of their worlds) and formal theories (deductive or speculative models or hypothetical representations seeking to explain practice of a field or discipline).

Practice knowledge depends on both artistry and science. That is, practice may be guided and shaped by theory, and may find its justifications in theory, but theory is not the sole cause and controller of the actions of professionals in their practice. Neither is practice comprehensively evidence-based. A considerable amount of practice has no scientific evidential base, in some cases because this evidence has not yet been identified and at times because, at least in principle, some aspects of professional practice can never be understood by the tools of empirical science. The latter is particularly so for most of the daily minute-by-minute decisions about each unique case. There are, however, other kinds of evidence for practice which can be found in professional craft knowledge and in the discussions and writing of professionals as practitioner researchers. Further, while we can illuminate the knowledge embedded in a piece of professional practice, there are some aspects of practice which cannot in principle ever be fully expressed in words. The term 'tacit knowledge' is used by Polanyi (1966) and Schön (1983) to describe such unknowable and inexpressible knowledge. We would argue, however, that there remains much of our practice which can be known and expressed in words if practitioners and researchers continue to seek to understand practice and find new tools for investigating, describing and measuring it. The use of 'tacit' to describe such knowledge is a loose and incorrect use of the term.

Disciplinary frameworks and paradigms

The traditions of the field or discipline in which individuals have been extensively educated profoundly determine their ways of seeing knowledge. Education within a discipline stamps us with particular views about the origins of knowledge, ways of seeing truth, what counts as evidence (ways of handling proof), views about theory and practice, views about appropriate means of achieving rigour. Even the meaning of rigour is disciplinarily determined. It is easy, when one is steeped in a particular way of seeing knowledge, to apply that approach unthinkingly to other kinds of knowledge (such as knowledge in another field of study) where it may not be appropriate or applicable.

Disciplinary frameworks are intimately connected with the philosophical position an individual adopts, and which we, perhaps unknowingly, bring to bear on our view of professional practice. They may inadvertently distort our understanding and our expectations of the practice if, for instance, we have taken a degree within a narrow subject field before joining a profession, or if we have extensively studied a particular discipline (e.g. music, physics) as a preparation for practice. For example, consider the comparison between knowing in the arts and in the sciences. Phenix (1964) defined six Realms of Meaning, expressing their nature with great clarity. They are Symbolics (language and mathematics); Empirics (the sciences of the physical world, of living things and of humans); Esthetics (the arts); Synnoetics (personal knowledge); Ethics (moral knowledge); and Synoptics (history, religion, philosophy).

While the fields of art and science are by no means mutually exclusive, since it is possible to find deep aesthetic meanings in things studied scientifically, and also to find scientific truth within aesthetic experiences, the key difference between them is in the kind of understanding gained. For scientists, it is empirical truth that they come to know (via observation and experimentation, which is then generalised). Science strives for objective certainties, and has particular ways of generating knowledge. This view, when brought into professional practice, causes unrealistic expectations, such as that there is objective knowledge of all aspects of practice 'out there' waiting to be discovered. By comparison, ways of knowing in the arts offer other perspectives on professional practice. Aesthetic meanings, Phenix wrote, are crucially concerned with particular and presented objects. The language of art (unlike science) is non-discursive, symbolical and metaphorical.

Successful artists in any field are people who think well with the characteristic materials of that field. Expertise in the arts grows out of prolonged experimentation with the materials, to exploit most fully their expressive possibilities. Thus, artists theorise in practice (Phenix 1964). The significance of a work of art depends on the manner in which the materials are organised into an organic unity whose form closely and significantly relates to its content. Evidence of the value of art relates to that piece of art and refers to aesthetic principles. The truth embodied in a piece of art is subtle, recognised by the response created in the audience, and may be perceived to be deeper and more enduring than that proposed in scientific laws. Some of the great art masterpieces or musical classics have stood the test of time and cultural differences. On the other hand, some scientific truths too have demonstrated considerable endurance.

Professional practitioners who are familiar with these very different ways of knowing are better equipped to see practice differently. For example, they would be able to recognise the essentially context-specific nature of 'good practice', and the importance of creating new knowledge in practice; they would recognise that the whole is more than the sum of the parts, and that competence is more than an agglomeration of competencies.

It is most important to recognise that there are different ways of sourcing, seeing, proving and conceptualising theory and practice. Across the different fields of knowledge there are also different ways of working rigorously. Most of us tend to bring one unquestioned way of seeing to our understanding of professional practice. We would do better to recognise and respect all the different ways of conceptualising knowledge. Thus equipped, we can move out from our one preferred, newly reviewed framework and become free to seek ways of understanding and developing knowledge in professional practice. As practitioners, we can then be ready to take our place in generating knowledge for our disciplines.

FRAMEWORKS FOR GENERATING KNOWLEDGE

When we seek to generate knowledge, we need to identify the questions we want to answer. We cannot know something that we have no way of ever asking a question about, and even to frame the question requires an understanding of what can be known.

The knower's philosophical stance

Knowledge is generated within different frames of reference. Different world views or *ontological perspectives* are an instance of this. While it is likely that individuals do not neatly fit or stay within any one ontological position, the perspectives we hold at a particular time will inform our knowledge generation. In particular, our ontological perspectives and assumptions underlie any theory or system of ideas we use to research and interpret the world.

The positivist/empiricist world view is one which sees the world as objective, independent of the knowers, and consisting of phenomena or events which are orderly and lawful. It dominates the field at present in physiotherapy and medicine. In these settings there has been a strong emphasis on the medical model and there is a strong valuing of visible and tangible evidence.

Other professions, such as occupational therapy and many areas of nursing, demonstrate a much greater emphasis on the social or human sciences. This is accompanied by a greater focus on the interpretive tradition (in which the world and reality are interpreted by people in the context of historical and social practices) and the critical perspective (in which there is a focus on the social world; people are socially located and therefore knowledge is always influenced by social interest). In these fields practice, and also its discourse, are alike imbued with notions of patient-centred care and recognition of the value of professional artistry.

A further frame of reference for knowledge generation is *epistemology*, in which questions are asked about 'the nature and derivation of knowledge, the scope of knowledge, and the reliability of claims to knowledge' (Flew 1984, p. 109). To positivists, for example, knowledge arises from the rigorous application of the scientific method and is measured against the criteria of objectivity, reliability and validity. For the positivist the only true knowledge is derived from empirical research using the scientific method. Commonly, such research remains silent on issues of ontology and epistemology, based on the assumption of an absolute (correct) position on the nature of reality and truth. In this tradition, evidence-based practice devotees recognise only propositional knowledge (derived from scientific research and theorisation) as justifiable evidence for practice.

Idealism, by comparison, arose in Germany in the late 19th century as a counter-movement to positivism. The idealist approaches of Dilthey (1833–1911) and Weber (1864–1920) focused on interpretive understanding (*verstehen*) as opposed to the explanatory and predictive approach of the physical sciences (*erklären*) (Smith 1983). Dilthey presented understanding as a hermeneutic process involving constant movement between parts and whole. This perspective results in a focus on human behaviour as occurring within a context, and the understanding or knowledge of human behaviour as requiring an understanding of this context.

Research paradigms

Research paradigms provide a framework for generating knowledge; they supply a particular shape and form to the truth which the generated knowledge proposition attempts to convey. Within a paradigm, assumptions, problems, research strategies, criteria and techniques are shared and taken for granted by a research community. Four distinct research paradigms can be identified as operating today.

The *empirico-analytical paradigm* is based on positivist philosophy and utilises the scientific method of observation and experiment in the empirical world, resulting in generalisations about the content and events of the world which can be used to predict future experience (Moore 1982). This paradigm is the basis for the medical model and the development of technical knowledge. Knowledge in this paradigm is discovered (i.e. universal and external truths are grasped) and justified on the basis of empirical processes which are reductionist, value-neutral, quantifiable, objective and operationalisable. Only those statements publicly verifiable by sense data are deemed valid.

The interpretive paradigm acknowledges local, multiple and specific constructed realities. Interpretive paradigm research seeks to interpret and generate knowledge of human phenomena in particular. The various research approaches in this paradigm (e.g. hermeneutics, ethnography, phenomenology) focus on the whole phenomenon under investigation, taking account of the context of the situation, the timings, the subjective meanings and intentions within the particular situation.

The critical paradigm generates emancipatory knowledge which enhances awareness of how our thinking is socially and historically constructed and how this limits our actions, in order to enable us to challenge these learned restrictions, compulsions or dictates of habit and to transform current structures, relationships and conditions that constrain development and reform. In this epistemology, knowledge is not grasped or discovered but is acquired through critical debate (Barnett 1990). The emancipatory tradition also focuses on the development of the individual, assuming that the process of becoming an adult requires critical thinking, reflecting upon the assumptions which underlie ideas and actions, and considering alternative ways of thinking (Brookfield 1987).

The artistic/holistic or *creative arts paradigm* (Fish 1998, Higgs & Titchen 2000), which builds on the ideas of Eliot Eisner (1985, 1993) is based on aesthetic, embodied, spiritual, intuitive and cognitive ways of knowing which occur in the practice of the creative arts. These ways of knowing have relevance to opening up a rich understanding of practice in a range of professional areas beyond the creative arts, including education for the caring professions (Fish 1998) and the health sciences (Benner 1984, Titchen 2000). Fish (1998) has argued that the development of professional artistry requires attention to certain dimensions of practice which are often invisible: the values, beliefs, attitudes, assumptions, expectations, feelings and knowledge lying below the surface and behind the actions of the practitioner.

CONCLUSION

In this chapter we have considered the nature, sources and contexts of practice knowledge. Recognising the primacy of practice, we have examined the nature of the practice context and acknowledged the influence of language and sociocultural historical perspectives on the way knowledge is viewed, created and used. We have explored various categorisations of practice knowledge and examined the importance of this knowledge within disciplinary frameworks and paradigms. We have concluded with consideration of different frameworks for generating knowledge and recommend that practitioners, educators and researchers learn to understand and value strategies for generating practice knowledge as they seek to extend their professional development, and to pursue quality in their professional practice.

To help readers reflect on their understanding of this complex topic we pose the following questions:

- How do you view practice knowledge? What forms of knowledge do you use in your practice? Which forms underlie your teaching? Which underlie and inform your research?

- What educational and research traditions formed part of your education? How have these influenced your world view and your view of what comprises knowledge?

- Which research paradigms have framed your own research and which have framed research reports of others that you have read? Within the framework of these paradigms, what sort of practice knowledge have you generated or acquired?

REFERENCES

Barnett, R. (1990). *The Idea of Higher Education*. Buckingham: Society for Research into Higher Education and Open University Press.
Benner, P. (1984). *From Novice to Expert: Excellence and Power in Clinical Nursing Practice*. Menlo Park, CA: Addison-Wesley.
Berlin, I. (1980). *Against the Current: Essays in the History of Ideas* (H. Hardy, ed.). London: Hogarth Press.
Berlin, I. (1990). *The Crooked Timber of Humanity*. Princeton, NJ: Princeton University Press.
Brookfield, S. D. (1987). *Developing Critical Thinkers*. Milton Keynes: Open University Press.
Carper, B. A. (1978). Fundamental patterns of knowing. *Advances in Nursing Science*, **1**, 13–23.
Eisner, E. W. (1985). *The Art of Educational Evaluation: A Personal View*. London: Falmer Press.
Eisner, E. W. (1993). Forms of understanding and the future of educational research. *Educational Researcher*, **22**(7), 5–11.
Eraut, M. (1994). *Developing Professional Knowledge and Competence*. London: Falmer Press.
Eraut, M. (2000). Non-formal learning and tacit knowledge in professional work. *British Journal of Educational Psychology*, **70**, 113–36.
Fish, D. (1998). *Appreciating Practice in the Caring Professions: Refocusing Professional Development and Practitioner Research*. Oxford: Butterworth-Heinemann.
Fish, D. & Coles, C. (eds) (1998). *Developing Professional Judgement in Health Care: Learning Through the Critical Appreciation of Practice*. Oxford: Butterworth-Heinemann.
Flew, A. (ed.) (1984). *A Dictionary of Philosophy*, 2nd edn. London: Pan.
Habermas, J. (1972). *Knowledge and Human Interest*. London: Heinemann.
Higgs, J. & Titchen, A. (1995). The nature, generation and verification of knowledge. *Physiotherapy*, **81**(9), 521–30.
Higgs, J. & Titchen, A. (2000). Knowledge and reasoning. In *Clinical Reasoning in the Health Professions*, 2nd edn (J. Higgs & M. Jones, eds) pp. 23–32. Oxford: Butterworth-Heinemann.
Higgs, J., Titchen, A. & Neville, V. (2001). Professional practice and knowledge. In *Practice Knowledge and Expertise in the Health Professions* (J. Higgs & A. Titchen, eds) pp. 3–9. Oxford: Butterworth-Heinemann.
Kennedy, M. (1987). Inexact sciences: professional education and the development of expertise. In *Review of Research in Education*, **14**, 133–68. Washington, DC.
MacIntyre, A. (1985). *After Virtue: A Study in Moral Theory*, 2nd edn. London: Duckworth.

Moore, T. W. (1982). *Philosophy of Education: An Introduction*. London: Routledge & Kegan Paul.

Phenix, P. H. (1964). *Realms of Meaning: A Philosophy of the Curriculum for General Education*. New York: McGraw-Hill.

Polanyi, M. (1958). *Personal Knowledge: Towards a Post-Critical Philosophy*. London: Routledge & Kegan Paul.

Polanyi, M. (1962). *Personal Knowledge*. London: Routledge & Kegan Paul.

Polanyi, M. (1966). *The Tacit Dimension*. Garden City, New York: Doubleday.

Reason, P. & Heron, J. (1986). Research with people: the paradigm of cooperative experiential enquiry. *Person-Centred Review*, **1**, 457–76.

Ryle, G. (1949). *The Concept of Mind*. Harmondsworth: Penguin Books.

Schein, E. (1973). *Professional Education*. New York: McGraw Hill.

Schön, D. A. (1983). *The Reflective Practitioner: How Professionals Think in Action*. New York: Basic Books.

Smith, J. K. (1983). Quantitative versus qualitative research: an attempt to clarify the issue. *Educational Researcher*, **12**, 6–13.

Stanford, M. (1998). *An Introduction to the Philosophy of History*. Oxford: Blackwell.

Titchen, A. (2000). *Professional Craft Knowledge in Patient-Centred Nursing and the Facilitation of its Development*. University of Oxford DPhil thesis. Oxford: Ashdale Press.

Torey, Z. (1999). *The Crucible of Consciousness: A Personal Exploration of the Conscious Mind*. Melbourne: Oxford University Press.

Wittgenstein, L. (1953/1997). *Philosophical Investigations*, 2nd edn, transl. G. E. Anscombe. Oxford: Blackwell.

5

Professions as communities of practice

Madeleine Abrandt Dahlgren,
Barbara Richardson and Björn Sjöström

INTRODUCTION

The perspective put forward in this chapter is that knowledge is socially and culturally constructed. The importance is emphasised of recognising the impact of the culturally grounded and shared values, beliefs and valid ways of reasoning within a profession. Learning to become a professional is thus not only a cognitive learning process but also a cultural learning process. It is argued that this cultural knowledge is just as essential as cognitive knowledge within a profession's practice knowledge base, and both forms of knowledge need to be made explicit among entry-level students, practitioners and researchers alike. Awareness of the cultural characteristics of a profession can contribute to the development of the knowledge base of the profession, in that it brings to the fore a dimension of professional knowledge that is seldom subjected to reflection and analysis. Knowing *about* the profession is considered as important as knowing *in* the profession, to understand the rationales for the ways of reasoning, acting and relating within the profession. Understanding one's profession can be considered a tool for enhanced awareness of the profession's specific contribution to solving problems. It can also be considered a tool for crossing boundaries and for collaboration between professions. The notion of professions as communities of practice and the emphasis on the cultural learning process could thus be seen as essential parts of the broader concept and process of professional socialisation.

KNOWLEDGE AS SOCIALLY AND CULTURALLY CONSTRUCTED

The general point of departure for this chapter is that knowledge is socially and culturally constructed. This means that being a member of a profession may be seen as participating in a specific social practice which is essential for shaping professional knowledge. Professional knowledge encompasses not only a certain body of cognitive knowledge, but also a set of shared values, beliefs, ways of reasoning and untold rules of thumb that characterise the field and that are constructed through the interaction and use of language between the professionals. This constructed (professional) knowledge is thus contextually grounded, being bound to a particular socio-cultural context. The learning process of becoming a professional is thus not only concerned with learning which phenomena are relevant to the specific profession and which factual knowledge is needed. The process is also a kind of cultural learning, comprising cognitive, practical and discursive aspects of knowing, being and doing in order to become a member of a professional community of practice. It is argued that awareness of the nature of this shared knowledge base is an important condition for professionals to be able to shape their professions for the future.

Having claimed the arguments in the previous paragraph, we position this chapter in a constructivist perspective on knowledge and knowledge formation. Constructivism is not a single theory, but rather a continuum of theories. There are, however, some characteristic features of the constructivist perspective on knowledge put forward in the literature (von Glasersfeld 1984, 1995, Doolittle 1999).

1. Knowledge is not passively accumulated but is the result of active cognition by the individual.
2. Cognition is an adaptive process that functions to make an individual's behaviour more viable in a particular environment.
3. Cognition organizes and makes sense of one's experience, and is not a process which renders an accurate representation of reality.
4. Knowing has roots in both biological/neurological construction and in social, cultural and language-based interactions (Doolittle 1999, p. 1).

This perspective opposes an objectivist or dualistic perspective on knowledge, which would encompass the notion of an external reality, separated from and knowable to the learner. In the cognitivist perspective, learning occurs when this external reality is represented in the mind of the learner. A social constructivist or non-dualistic perspective instead emphasises social interaction as the process moulding individual conceptions into a shared knowledge base. Through this process, individuals appropriate as well as contribute their individual knowledge. Thus learning cannot be understood without considering the mutually transforming process that social interaction brings about. There is no objective knowledge independent of human beings as knowers; people are always interpreting what is to be learned from the contextual circumstances in which they live. In this sense, learning is situated in a specific context. This description of the constructivist perspective can be viewed as a bridge between cognitive and sociocultural theories. Billet (1996) has argued that cognitive and sociocultural theories are complementary in a number of aspects, that the two literatures can be bridged in a way that is sympathetic to both theories, and that this helps to understand more thoroughly the nature of situated learning. The overlapping areas where the two theories address similar aspects (Billet 1996) are as follows:

- Expertise is domain-specific. There is no universal expertise that can be applied across all fields. Situationally dependent understanding, rule-based concepts and knowledge of procedures are paramount for the expert.
- Knowledge is constructed through problem-solving. The links between problem-solving and socially determined, goal-directed activity point to the construction of knowledge, embedded in the social circumstances where knowledge is appropriated.
- Compilation of knowledge is negotiated in social circumstances as indicated above. The requirements and characteristics of particular social circumstances contribute to individuals' highly automated (highly practised and instantaneously applied) procedures (Billet 1996, p. 268).
- Transfer of knowledge is socially and culturally constructed. Transfer is the ability to apply knowledge in a novel situation. Transfer is not only the product of internal mechanisms, but is dependent on the individual's ability to respond to particular conditions under which the knowledge to be transferred is constructed.
- Individuals' efforts are related to social practice, individual dispositions and what is privileged in social practice, rather than being universal and predictable outcomes as a response to given stimuli.
- Socially determined dispositional factors are relational to cognitive structures and activities. Dispositions are inherent in the co-construction, organisation and deployment of cognitive structures. Dispositions originate in both personal histories and cultural circumstances.

It has been argued that professional knowledge is contextually grounded. What, then, is meant by the concept 'context' from the particular perspective we are pursuing here? The term is derived from the Latin *contextus*, the past participle of *contextere*, which means to weave together or join together (Scharfstein 1989). Context is that which surrounds or environs the object of our inquiry and helps, by its relevance, to explain it. The environment may be of any sort: temporal, geographical, cultural, cognitive, emotional, etc. (ibid., p. 1). In a sociocultural perspective, context is not something external that affects us; it is part of our understanding and is not separable from the process of giving meaning to the object of inquiry (Säljö 2000). This means that a situation is understood in terms of the phenomena involved, and, conversely, we are aware of the phenomena from the perspective of the specific situation. The ways people learn and understand are thus dependent on the cultural circumstances under which they live. Understanding requires a familiarity with cultural traditions and communicative patterns.

The sociocultural perspective on learning, thinking and action thus focuses on how individuals and groups acquire physical and cognitive resources and on the interplay between the collective and the individual level (Säljö 2000, p. 18). According to Säljö, the interplay between the collective and individual levels refers to what can be achieved in a culture and what single members can capture, how the collective knowledge is reproduced in individuals, and what parts of the collective knowledge the individual will master. More directly put, the assumptions regarding the relationships between the different levels of knowing in practice involve an interaction between the local and the global level. This can be illustrated via Wenger's (1998) discussion and interpretation of the concepts *meaning*, *practice*, *community* and *identity*.

SOCIAL PARTICIPATION AS A PROCESS OF LEARNING

According to Wenger (1998), in order to characterise social participation as a process of learning and knowing it is important to emphasise four essential components of this process. *Meaning* is a way of talking about the individual and the collective ability of the group to experience the world as meaningful. *Practice* is a way of talking about the shared historical and social resources, frameworks and perspectives that are important for action within a culture. *Community* is defined as a 'way of talking about the social configurations in which our enterprises are defined as worth pursuing and our participation is recognisable as competence' (ibid., p. 5). *Identity* is a way of talking about how learning changes the learner and creates personal histories of becoming in the context of communities. These four concepts are deeply interconnected and are mutually defining, according to Wenger.

Looking closely at a professional encounter within health care, the relationships between the four concepts could be interpreted as described in the following. The *meaning* aspect refers to the features of the health care situation that stand out as salient and meaningful to the professional. It is reasonable to assume that (for example) a nurse, a doctor or a physiotherapist would focus on somewhat different aspects of the situation and consider them the most important features to attend to. Knowledge about these features thus gives information about how the situation is contextualised and defined from the perspective of the professional practitioner.

The meaning aspect is thereby related to the *practice* aspect, which would refer to the shared agreement (between practitioners) about suitable actions to take in the particular case. In today's era of evidence-based practice there might be conflicting messages of what the shared agreement is. Should the practitioner base decisions about the actions to take on prevailing traditions, on recommendations derived from research, or is there a middle ground where an analysis of the particular case would be appraised against the research recommendations (which might be rejected in favour of the individual needs of the client)? Later in this chapter we give an empirical example of how nurses reason when they are assessing acute postoperative pain, illustrating the way different knowledge bases for action are used in the clinical situation (Sjöström 1995).

The practice aspect is also closely linked to the *community* aspect. The social configurations in which our practices operate help to define expectations regarding practitioners' competence. Simultaneously, the community aspect also defines the boundaries of the knowledge claims for a specific profession. Professions might have conflicting conceptions about claims for certain fields of knowledge, and in times of economical constraints this disparity might be even more accentuated as professions strive to legitimise their existence within the health care system.

Finally, the *identity* concept is related to knowledge of all the previous aspects. The individual's identity as a professional is achieved when the individual has developed understanding and capacities related to the meaning, practice and community dimensions of professional socialisation, and has appropriated these. These knowledges might be more or less explicit or function tacitly in the individual professional, and might appear earlier or later in the educational process. It is even reasonable to assume that, for some, the feeling of identity within a specific profession does not appear until after some years of experience.

LEARNING AS PERSONAL, INTERPERSONAL AND COMMUNITY PROCESSES

A sociocultural perspective on learning and development has also been described by Rogoff (1995), who suggested that such a perspective incorporates three planes of description and analysis, focusing on *personal, interpersonal* and *community* processes. Rogoff does not suggest that these processes are hierarchical or separate entities; on the contrary, they are viewed as inseparable. Processes on all planes are always interrelated and integrated in sociocultural activity, but one plane may be foregrounded and the others backgrounded as we focus on one or the other.

The metaphor given by Rogoff (1995) for describing learning processes on a personal plane is *participatory appropriation*. This refers to how individuals change through their involvement in sociocultural activity. Through participation, individuals change and transform their ways of understanding and handling a situation, so that they are prepared for handling later, similar situations through their previous experiences. Rogoff claims that the concept of appropriation should be distinguished from the concept of internalisation. The two concepts represent two different theoretical perspectives, she argues. The appropriation perspective emphasises development as a dynamic, mutual process, involving people's active participation in cultural activities. The internalisation perspective views development in terms of a static, bounded acquisition or transmission of pieces of knowledge.

Learning processes on the interpersonal plane are viewed by Rogoff (1995) as *guided participation*. This learning emphasises the mutual involvement of individuals and how they communicate and coordinate their involvement with materials and arrangements collaboratively managed by themselves and their peers, as they participate in 'socio-culturally structured collective activities' (p. 147). Research focusing on this plane has been directed towards the system of interpersonal engagements and arrangements that are involved in participation in social learning activities.

Rogoff (1995) uses the metaphor *apprenticeship* to describe how learning and development occur in the community plane. The metaphor extends the idea of craftsmanship, Rogoff claims, since it incorporates all kinds of culturally organised activity in which individuals participate. The concept of apprenticeship here refers to the system of values that guides the newcomer into a community of practice, the relationship between the nature of the activity involved and the institutions of the community in which it occurs.

In a sociocultural perspective, as described by Säljö (2000), the Vygotskian terms *psychological tools* (see Vygotsky 1978) or, as Säljö calls them, *discursive tools*, are important. Discursive tools refer to the intellectual and physical tools that we use when we understand our surrounding world or when we act in it. Discursive tools can be artefacts constructed by people and through which knowledge is mediated. The individual can use a calculator, for example, without having to know all the programming that has been put into the tool. The tools pertaining to a culture are simultaneously intellectual and practical in their nature and should not be regarded as separate entities isolated from the culture. The simultaneous intellectual and practical nature of the discursive tools is based in a non-dualistic perspective of practice under which manual activities are not thoughtless and mental activities are not disembodied.

The kinds of knowledge and skills that constitute discursive tools emanate from the insights and patterns of actions that are built up historically in a community of practice and into which we become socialised through interaction with other people. From a sociocultural point of view, the issue of learning is thus a question of achieving the resources necessary for thinking and accomplishing practical projects that are part of our culture and our surrounding world. In all these processes, the decisive feature is communication between people. It is through communication that sociocultural resources are created, but it is also through communication that they are reproduced. The processes described above (i.e. learning as personal, interpersonal and community activity) must be recognised as an essential part of practice knowledge, important to make explicit in the learning process as well as among practitioners and researchers. They could also be used as analytical tools for the description and enhancement of the professional knowledge base in the health care professions.

LEARNING IN PRACTICE – AN EMPIRICAL EXAMPLE OF NURSES' AND PHYSICIANS' ASSESSMENT OF POSTOPERATIVE PAIN

In the following section we illustrate theory concerning professions as communities of practice with some empirical results from a study (Sjöström 1995) which aimed to describe the content, development and credibility of experienced nurses' and physicians' clinical reasoning and acting in a common and, for the patient, problematic situation. The example is chosen from the field of pain assessment. It is known from the literature that about 75% of patients who have undergone surgery report moderate to severe postoperative pain (Donovan et al 1987, Ketovuori 1987, Carr & Thomas 1997). Despite the development of new medical techniques, new drugs and pain management programmes, the reported incidence is surprisingly stable. The results of this study describe nurses' and physicians' ways of thinking in pain assessment and can contribute to understanding the learning aspects of clinical know-how, which can be seen as a part of the *meaning* and *practice* aspects of Wenger's (1998) learning model.

Participants in the study were 30 nurses and 30 physicians, both more and less experienced. Semistructured interviews were used, comprising a number of questions relevant to the investigation which the participants could answer freely. In addition, the nurses and physicians carried out pain ratings on patients using a visual analogue scale (VAS) of how the patients experienced their pain postoperatively. This scale is commonly used in pain research. To study the credibility of the participants' knowing, the ways of reasoning were related to how congruent the practitioners' and the patients' ratings were on the scale.

The data collection focused on the procedures used in the pain assessment by the participants, the initial interview encompassing previous experience and professional role, including personal attitudes to postoperative care. The participant physicians and nurses both followed the procedure described here. After the initial interview the postoperative patients in pain indicated their present pain on a 10-cm baseline VAS. Thereafter, a participant met each patient and carried out a pain assessment in accordance with normal routines (i.e. not using a scale). The researcher observed the pain assessment. After leaving the room the participant was asked to rate the patient's pain on a VAS. The rating of the pain score was followed by a second interview which focused in detail on the participant's perception of the patient's situation. This was followed by questions about how and on what basis the participant judged the patient's pain. The following approach was used: Give a short description of the patient, his or her situation, feelings and pain. How much pain (intensity/type) does the patient experience? How did you come to that conclusion? What role did your clinical experience play? Three different postoperative patients were assessed by each participant nurse and physician respectively. Finally, a more extensive interview was conducted, concerning general conceptions of pain management and the significance of experience. All the interviews were audio-taped and later transcribed verbatim.

The results showed that the nurses and physicians used different assessment criteria for deciding on the patients' level of pain. One strategy for assessing patients' pain was dependent upon *how the patient looks*. This strategy for assessing pain contained two main directions: signs which were more general, such as body movements and grimaces and signs which more specifically indicated clinical state, such as heart rate, pupil size, skin characteristics, the flow of tears, as illustrated in the following quote:

> *Participant:* You look at her, she's not so ... she's so contactable and she's so alert. She can talk with me. She doesn't have any tachycardia, she doesn't have high blood pressure, she isn't vasoconstricted and, basically, she looks fresh and nice, and she says that she's not in that much pain. But it ... she seemed quite unaffected, both as regards circulation and respiration. Her skin is warm.

Another strategy was to assess the pain according to *what the patient says*. The focus here was on the content of the verbal communication. The category also implies that the patient was approached with the intention of communicating. This is exemplified by the dialogue below:

> *Participant:* She asked for pain relief herself.
>
> *Interviewer:* And then ... then you gave ... ?
>
> *Participant:* Yes, I think it's the patient one should listen to primarily.

The third strategy for assessing pain was to follow *the patient's way of talking*. In this category, interest focuses on the form of the communication rather than the actual content, i.e. how the patient looks when communicating.

> *Participant:* Well, if he ... you could say, how he expresses himself in relation to his appearance at the time. I combine them in some way. And ... because I mean, there are those who you can see are in incredible pain but they say, 'No, but I'm not in any particular pain'. And then they are anyway.

The final pain assessment strategy was to rely on *past experience of similar circumstances*. Experience is central in this category, and it has a number of themes: the staff members have 'seen it before', or they claim to know that certain groups of patients are in pain, and that the level of anxiety has an influence. The focus is not on the individual patient but rather on how patients with certain diagnoses, undergoing certain types of surgery and having certain types of anaesthesia usually experience pain:

> *Participant:* Well, [it was a] major operation, and, well, that she ... even if she didn't show that she was in such great pain, so she seems a bit more ... it wasn't this sort of calm and harmonious, rather she was embarrassed by all this and it was difficult and so she ...
>
> *Interviewer:* What is most important to you when you assess her?
>
> *Participant:* Well, it was probably the long operation and that two large incisions had been made in two places.

Distribution of assessment criteria categories and group comparisons

The frequencies of the four identified criteria categories used in the pain assessment are presented in Table 5.1. The categories do not describe the ability to assess postoperative pain hierarchically, but rather constitute a consistent and contextually grounded description of the broad variation of the practitioners' ways of assessing pain.

As can be seen from the table, the assessment criteria categories *How the patient looks* and *What the patient says* clearly dominated for nurses as well as for physicians. Nurses referred somewhat more often to *Past experience* than physicians, while physicians more often than nurses considered *The patient's way of talking*.

Another focus of the study was to investigate the role of experiential learning for the chosen assessment strategies. Four categories of experience stood out. In the first category, *I have learnt a typology of patients*, experience meant having seen the totality, that is, the progress of a normal case after a certain type of operation, a certain type of anaesthesia and the usual degree of pain of these patients as well as how much pain relief they require and tolerate. Experience had established models which were used for a standardised classification of patients. The concept of typology is regarded as a

Table 5.1 Distribution of criteria categories for pain assessment among staff members in per cent and absolute numbers of statements ($n = 170$)

Criteria	All staff members		Nurses		Physicians	
	%	n	%	n	%	n
How the patient looks	50	85	51	45	49	40
What the patient says	41	71	42	37	40	34
The patient's way of talking	5	7	1	1	9	6
Past experience	4	7	6	5	2	2
Total	100	170	100	88	100	82

(From Sjöström (1995), with permission of Acta Universitatis Gothoburgensis.)

good description of this category but it is understood in a broader sense which includes what is common, what is special and what is different:

> *Participant:* Well, I have a clear picture of what these patients usually look like. I know that in her case, well, she behaves like they usually do.
>
> *Interviewer:* When you say that you have a clear picture of how these patients usually act, what do you mean?
>
> *Participant:* Well, laparotomies, I mean. That was what she went through. If you've made a fairly small incision in the intestine.

The second category of experiential learning was *I have learnt to listen to the patients*. This category focused on patients' verbal communication for criteria of the assessment, experience having shown that pain is an individual phenomenon and that the patient is the only one who can decide whether he/she is in pain or not:

> *Participant:* Well, it's taught me that if the patient only says I'm in pain, then I have to reckon that she is in pain. It's her experience of it, but then I also have to include it in my assessment …

I have learnt what to look for was the third category discerned in the interviews. In this category, experience refers to the assessment process by describing what to refer to when assessing pain. Experience influences and reformulates the process of assessment by recognising new criteria and by combining different assessment criteria:

> *Participant:* Well, above all to narrow down the problem from the periphery, so that you don't spoil the picture by being too fussy and disturbing the patient unnecessarily, so to say.
>
> *Interviewer:* You mean, that you began …
>
> *Participant:* I began by looking at the patient and seeing if she had … I mean, you can often see if a patient is lying there and in pain, and then he doesn't look calm and rosy and half asleep, relaxed. Now she didn't in fact have any monitoring connected, but one could also check pressure and pulse. But with an eye on when … on the chart you also cast a glance at when you walk past, then you see that it's calm and peaceful and there are no signs of there being any excessive pain there.

The fourth category was *I have learnt what to do for the patient*. Here, assessment was seen as a part of a whole which included the pain treatment as well. Experience is oriented towards the possibilities of medical treatment regarding both what to do and how to do it. The assessment is seen as integrated with and not separated from the treatment:

> *Participant:* Well, that you … don't hesitate to give pain relief, and that you don't need to be afraid that they'll suffer from a whole lot of after-effects as a result. Because I've learnt to look after this sort of patient and I've … you learn that it's never … well, I shouldn't say this, but it is most often never wrong to give, while it is wrong not to give. Like you can often be afraid in the beginning because it's so much … Now, the thing is that they are supposed to go home

sometimes. Then ... Voltarol Supp., but I don't think it helps in the case of such an operation, I don't think so.

Table 5.2 Distribution of experience-associated categories for pain assessment among nurses and physicians ($n = 161$)

Category of experience	Nurses		Physicians	
	%	n	%	n
A typology of patients	42	35	53	41
To listen to patients	10	8	12	9
What to look for	15	13	17	13
What to do for the patient	33	28	18	14
Total	100	84	100	77

(From Sjöström (1995), with permission of Acta Universitatis Gothoburgensis.)

A summary of the distribution of the statements over the different experience categories is presented in Table 5.2. As can be seen, the category *I have learnt a typology of patients* was the most common category for both groups. Nurses more than physicians focused on what to do for patients. Physicians relied most heavily on their knowledge of patient typologies.

Congruence of pain ratings between patients' and practitioners' ratings on VAS and impact of professional role and experience on accuracy of pain assessment

A comparison between physicians and nurses showed that the pain scores of both groups deviated from (were less than) the patients' ratings and that the deviation increased with higher levels of pain as reported by patients (Table 5.3). Physicians' pain scores (of patient pain) were closer to those of the patients than were the nurses'. The relationships between practitioners' experience and deviation of the pain scores from those of the patients are summarised in Table 5.4.

The highest deviation from patients' ratings was found among *very experienced* nurses (-2.0) and the smallest deviation was found among *less experienced* and *very experienced* physicians ($-0.8; p < 0.05$). Thus, increasing experience did not seem to have an impact on the accuracy of the physicians' assessment, while there was a tendency towards increasing deviation from the patients' ratings among more experienced nurses.

The coefficients indicated that increasing clinical experience resulted in more consistent pain ratings, earlier for physicians than for nurses. Furthermore, in the case of experienced nurses, these more consistent pain ratings were associated with a systematic underestimation.

Table 5.3 Mean and standard deviation (SD) of nurses' and physicians' deviation from patients' ratings ($n = 60$)

Patients' ratings	Nurses			Physicians		
	n	Mean	SD	n	Mean	SD
<4.5	3	0	0.7	0		
4.5–5.4	5	−1.1	1.1	9	−0.4	1.1
5.5–6.4	9	−1.3	1.3	12	−0.9	1.0
6.5–7.4	7	−1.7	1.0	7	−1.3	1.2
>7.5	6	−2.6	1.0	2	−1.8	2.1

(From Sjöström (1995), with permission of Acta Universitatis Gothoburgensis.)

Table 5.4 Distribution of the deviation from patients' ratings distributed among subgroups ($n = 60$)

Rating deviation	Nurses			Physicians		
	LE	E	VE	LE	E	VE
Mean	−1.6	−1.0	−2.0	−0.8	−1.1	−0.8
SD	1.1	1.2	1.2	1.5	0.9	1.1
n	5	14	11	7	9	14

LE, less experienced; E, experienced; VE, very experienced.
(From Sjöström (1995), with permission of Acta Universitatis Gothoburgensis.)

Accuracy of different strategies in pain assessment

A combination of experience and assessment criteria categories underlie pain assessment strategies. Strategies may vary between as well as within individuals when carrying out pain assessment. We focus here on the question of the relative efficacy of different strategies, defined as the discrepancy (in VAS scores) between the pain ratings of the patients and the practitioners. Hence, an overview of the mean discrepancies as well as absolute frequencies of occurrence of the various strategies is provided in Table 5.5.

The most common strategy, *I have learnt a typology of patients* and *How the patient looks*, resulted in a fairly high discrepancy of 1.9 VAS scores from the patients' own ratings. The strategy *I have learnt to listen to patients* and *What the patient says* resulted in the significantly ($p < 0.05$, t-test) smallest discrepancy (0.7 VAS scores).

With this example of empirical research, we emphasise that the availability of descriptions of how a group of people use perception in professional settings is in itself a resource for enhancing awareness. The primary value of an analysis of the kind presented here is thus that the description of categories may be fed into basic and further education of staff in health care. A prerequisite for the development of professional competence is an awareness of one's strong and weak points. Description of people's ways of reasoning is thus a fruitful tool for learning. The accuracy of categorisation of a single subject is of minor importance compared to the category system itself. According to Kim (1996, p. 115):

> Knowledge regarding practitioners' personal theories and how they are applied in specific situations is of utmost importance since the quality of nursing practice depends critically on the nature of nurses' personal theories and their application.

Table 5.5 The outcome of the different pain assessment strategies given as mean discrepances between visual analogue scale scorings by patients and staff members

Experience	Criteria	Mean discrepancy	Number
I have learnt a typology of patients	How the patient looks	1.9	41
	What the patient says	1.4	28
	The patient's way of talking	2	2
	Past experience of similar circumstances	1	4
I have learnt to listen to the patient	How the patient looks	2.5	4
	What the patient says	0.7	11
	The patient's way of talking	2	1
	Past experience of similar circumstances	5	1
I have learnt what to look for	How the patient looks	2.4	14
	What the patient says	2.1	10
	The patient's way of talking	1	2
	Past experience of similar circumstances	N/A	N/A
I have learnt what to do for the patient	How the patient looks	1.8	19
	What the patient says	1.3	18
	The patient's way of talking	2	3
	Past experience of similar circumstances	2.5	2

(From Sjöström (1995), with permission of Acta Universitatis Gothoburgensis.)

What health practitioners discern from a clinical situation can be seen as an intentional act influenced by the rules and values of the social and cultural discourse considered as a functional way of perceiving this problem. The results of this study show, however, that what is discerned and how the clinical situation is experienced varied among the practitioners.

The nurses underestimated the patients' pain more than the physicians did, and the group that did this the most were the most experienced nurses. The results also showed that they had learned by experiential learning systematically to underestimate patients' experience of pain. The underestimation was greater, the more pain the patients reported. Another finding, when relating the qualitative categories to the ratings of pain, was that the most frequent category (based on theoretical learning) deviated most from the patients' ratings. The category comprising a patient-oriented perspective deviated least from the patients' ratings.

The study made it possible to identify different ways of approaching clinical problems, and by combining these with the patients' perspectives (in this case, VAS ratings), the research demonstrated the practical consequences of different ways of assessing patients' pain. The implication is that if practitioners continue to use certain unreflected ways of approaching the problem, the incidence of reported postoperative pain will remain unchanged. The results also indicate that learning from experience does not necessarily mean only gaining knowledge about how things usually are, but also that learning that patients and conditions may vary. Experience thus may be one means of understanding the range of normal and abnormal conditions.

IMPLICATIONS FOR EDUCATION

Embracing a perspective of constructivism acknowledges that knowledge is bound to sociocultural contexts and is socially constructed. This is a powerful message to teach health care students. However, although it can encourage them to have confidence in actions for which they are able to provide adequate reasons, they also need to be aware of the power biases in cultural practices which can result in their views as individuals being overwhelmed by the weight of stronger collective views, and for opportunities for progress to be lost. It is of paramount importance for students to appreciate the ways in which they as individuals contribute to a prevailing culture, the processes through which cultural behaviour is established, and how they can influence the development of the professional knowledge base.

Understanding of one's own profession is also a tool for understanding other professions, a tool for crossing boundaries between professions (Wenger 1998). It has been argued that knowledge is bound to a specific sociocultural practice, but there is also broader discourse which helps to negotiate across practices what is considered to be knowledge. This broader discourse is necessary for development, and could be ignored if knowledge is made totally practice-specific. Wenger reminds us that what is counted as knowledge is also a matter of the positions of our practices with respect to the broader historical, social and institutional discourses and styles to which people orient their practices and by which they legitimise their knowledge claims. It is thus necessary for reflection about learning in a community of practice to incorporate encounters with other perspectives as well as those prevailing in a specific practice, to cross the boundaries between communities of practice.

Culture is thought to hide 'more than it reveals, and strangely enough, what it hides it hides most effectively from its own participants' (Hall 1959). Culture is regarded as the acquired knowledge people use to interpret their experiences and generate behaviour (Spradley 1980). It is created, defined and altered (Charon 1995) by people and can be inferred, not observed, through behaviour (Wolcott 1988). A critical understanding and awareness of ways in which the collective thinking, behaviour and beliefs of a group of practitioners leads to a collective construction of their working practices can give students insight into how their individual behaviour can both shape and be shaped by that culture. It can also provide them with insight into how a collective view of work practice can impact upon the way their professional knowledge is utilised and generated in that work context.

Professional health care knowledge is constructed by health care professionals as they integrate their procedural and propositional knowledge with experiential knowledge gained from their work with patients/clients and other health care staff. In the workplace practitioners gain an understanding of the perceived relevance of their work practices; they will adopt or appropriate, as Rogoff (1995) suggests, the attitudes to and behaviours of work that they see valued by their peers. This interplay between an individual's knowledge and understanding of practice and the perceived recognition of it by others in a health care group will influence the ways in which individuals utilise their knowledge in patient care and in their interactions with others in a health care team. This in turn will reinforce that aspect of working practice, increasing the chances of its being repeated on future occasions.

The writing of Giddens (1982) suggests that it is through such processes that the social world of practice of health care becomes meaningful to practitioners. According to Giddens, a working practice culture is continuously constructed and reconstructed through the social structures of the interactions which take place in a clinical setting: people's activities contribute to their culture and this is reproduced in their tacit understanding of 'knowing how to behave'. Consciously or unconsciously, practitioners will gain a state of 'knowledgeability' about what is collectively known about their departmental practices and the conditions of their behaviour within it. This occurs through tacit modes of knowing in which the routine features of everyday behaviour are recognised. Powerful cultural messages can thus be perpetuated, reinforced and promulgated in behaviour that tacitly and uncritically accepts the credibility of current practice. As Giddens (p. 37) declared, 'The most minor or trivial forms of social action are tied to structural properties of the overall society and to the coalescence of institutions over long stretches of historical time'. Importantly, the social theory he puts forward assumes that people can do otherwise. In accordance with this theory, practitioners are able to make themselves both the subject and the object of their awareness.

This argument emphasises the central concern for students to appreciate that what practitioners do today will be reinforced and regurgitated by practitioners tomorrow, thus limiting development of professional knowledge and professional activities, unless they take a critical and analytical stance to ensure consciously that their actions befit their purpose. The responsibility for establishing this way of looking at practice rests particularly with academic and clinical educators. Cognition is distributed over mind and body, the activity and the culturally organised setting (Lave 1988, p. 1). Students learn all the time, but professional learning is facilitated by educators taking part of a student's learning process and sharing examples from the experience of their life, to create thinking patterns which will gather to formulate a professional paradigm. This process is sometimes referred to as providing the scaffolding of orientation to the task (Rogoff 1990, p. 93). It is important for educators to accept that individual knowledge construction is essentially grounded in experiential knowledge. Students will learn propositional and procedural knowledge in common with other students of a profession, but it is the experiential processes of integrating that knowledge in a professional context which will dominate the development of their individual professional knowledge base.

The importance of experiential knowledge has been gaining recognition in notions of learning which stretch from novice to expert performance (Benner 1984, Dreyfus & Dreyfus 1986). Novices are categorised as displaying 'context-free' skills, advanced beginners as showing an ability to incorporate situational aspects of work. This characterisation has led to educational strategies which promote a notion of incremental skill learning which ignores the potency of processes of scaffolding and participatory appropriation (i.e. how individuals change through their involvement in sociocultural activity and transform their ways of understanding and handling a situation (Rogoff 1990)). There are benefits in trying to analyse the components of professional practice but there are accompanying dangers in assuming that they must then be taught to students in similar packages of knowledge. Stimuli to learning are not separate from the process of doing activities (Lave 1988, p. 171), nor can they be broken into single components, as might be inferred from textbook attempts to describe stages of propositional learning. Because of the tacit nature of experiential knowledge and the complexity of its formulation in the development of an individual's thinking patterns, it cannot be predicted and controlled by predefined educational processes. However, repeated and recurrent professional experiences which contain rich contextual cues for professional action can do much to embed a strong sense of the qualities of being a professional.

This presents a challenge to curricula in which knowledge and skills are learned in the decontextualised context of the classroom, with the expectation that students will be able simply to transfer this learning to the real world of practice. The crucial point is that students' learning occurs throughout their whole experience: through the multitude of pervasive covert and overt innuendo, gestures, behaviour, verbalising and dress which are part of the profession's culture, whether in the classroom or the clinic or other workplace. The task facing educators is to ensure that students gain an awareness of the cultural sea which embraces the classroom and the clinic in which students' professional paradigms are formed. This can be done by adopting an educational approach which is focused on providing students with experiences which develop their insight into the complex, fluid, human situations of practice and which enable them to act wisely, grounded in an awareness of self as an active agent (Elliot 1991, p. 130). A concept of a community of practice which extends from the classroom to the workplace emphasises a continuity of learning which mirrors the continual flux and change of practice settings. An understanding of the processes through which professional knowledge continually develops is the basis for the development of behaviour which continually challenges the 'being and doing' of practice, rather than merely knowing facts about it. This conative dimension of a personal disposition to taking professional action and adopting the behaviour of a professional is essential. Competence in learning new knowledge and skills is lost without the 'hearts and minds' (Osler 1913) commitment inherent in a professional manner.

Development of professional knowledge is intrinsic to principles of a continuous quality improvement of care that is currently adopted by many health care services globally. The managed care concept of the USA (Weiner et al 2002) and clinical governance policies of the UK (Moores 1999) both focus on a culture of accountability and audit of working practices. These practices are underpinned by a commitment to the recognition and sharing of good practice which will foster improvements in the allocation of health care resources and in the organisation and processes of care (Wilcock 1998). A disposition in professionals to appraise current practice in relation to their own ideals and ambitions will help develop confidence in their professional judgements. A vigour of propensity towards professional action will be driven by a confident professional identification, born of a clear understanding of competence and autonomy legitimised by the professional peer group. There is an increasing gap between education and practice; between the academic values of educational institutes and service requirements and consumer expectations (Garcia-Barbero 1995). If students gain an understanding of the powerful influences exerted by working cultures on their practice, they can more easily take a critical stance relative to the activities in their workplaces, acknowledging their ability to contribute not only to the development of their professional practice knowledge but also to the professional knowledge base at large.

REFERENCES

Benner, P. (1984). *From Novice to Expert: Excellence and Power in Clinical Nursing Practice.* Menlo Park, CA: Addison-Wesley.
Billet, S. (1996). Situated learning: bridging socio-cultural and cognitive theorising. *Learning and Instruction*, 6(3), 263–80.
Carr, E. C. J. & Thomas, V. J. (1997). Anticipating and experiencing post-operative pain: the patients' perspective. *Journal of Clinical Nursing*, 6, 191–201.
Charon, J. M. (1995). *Symbolic Interactionism: An Introduction, an Interpretation, an Integration*, 5th edn. Englewood Cliffs, NJ: Simon and Schuster.
Donovan, M., Dillon, P. & McGuire, L. (1987). Incidence and characteristics of pain in a sample of medical–surgical inpatients. *Pain*, 30, 69–78.

Doolittle, P. (1999). *Constructivism and Online Education*. Paper presented at online conference on Teaching Online in Higher Education. Available at http://www.tandl.vt.edu/doolittle/research/tohe1999/types.html.

Dreyfus, H. L. & Dreyfus, S. E. (1986). *Mind Over Machine – The Power of Human Intuition and Expertise in the Era of the Computer*. Oxford: Blackwell.

Elliot, J. (1991). *Action Research for Educational Change*. Milton Keynes: Open University Press.

Garcia-Barbero, M. (1995). Medical education in light of the World Health Organisation Health for All Strategy and the European Union. *Medical Education*, **29**, 3–12.

Giddens, A. (1982). *Profiles and Critiques in Social Theory*. London: Macmillan Press.

Hall, E. T. (1959). *The Silent Language*. New York: Anchor Books, Doubleday.

Ketovuori, H. (1987). Nurses and patients' conceptions of wound pain and the administration of analgesics. *Journal of Pain and Symptom Management*, **2**, 213–18.

Kim, S. (1996). Fakultetsopponenten sammanfattar [The faculty opponent summarises]. *Pedagogisk Forskning i Sverige [Educational Research in Sweden]*, **2**, 112–15.

Lave, J. (1988). *Cognition in Practice, Mind, Mathematics and Culture in Everyday Life*. Cambridge, MA: Cambridge University Press.

Moores, Y. (1999). Clinical governance and nursing. *Professional Nurse*, **15**(2), 74–5.

Osler, W. (1913). Examination, examiners and examinees. *Lancet*, Oct. 11, 1047–50.

Rogoff, B. (1990). *Apprenticeship in Thinking: Cognitive Development in Social Context*. New York: Oxford University Press.

Rogoff, B. (1995). Observing socio-cultural activity on three planes: participatory appropriation, guided participation, and apprenticeship. In *Socio-Cultural Studies of Mind*, (J. V. Wertsch, ed.) pp. 139–64. Cambridge: Cambridge University Press.

Säljö, R. (2000). *Kunskap i Praktiken [Knowledge in Practice]*. Stockholm: Prisma.

Scharfstein, B. (1989). *The Dilemma of Context*. New York: New York University Press.

Sjöström, B. (1995). *Assessing Acute Postoperative Pain: Assessment Strategies and Quality in Relation to Clinical Experience and Professional Role*. Doctoral thesis. Göteborg: Acta Universitatis Gothoburgensis; vol. 98.

Spradley, J. P. (1980). *Participant Observation*. New York: Holt, Rinehart and Winston.

von Glasersfeld, E. (1984). An introduction to radical constructivism. In *The Invented Reality* (P. Watzlawick, ed.) pp. 17–40. New York: Norton.

von Glasersfeld, E. (1995). A constructivist approach to teaching. In *Constructivism in Education* (L. P. Steffe & J. Gale, eds) pp. 3–16. Hillsdale, NJ: Erlbaum.

Vygotsky, L. S. (1978). *Mind in Society: The Development of Higher Psychological Process*. Cambridge, MA: Harvard University Press.

Weiner, J., Gillam, S. & Lewis, R. (2002). Organization and financing of British primary care groups and trusts: observations through the prism of US managed care. *Journal of Health Services Research and Policy*, **7**(1), 43–50.

Wenger, E. (1998). *Communities of Practice: Learning, Meaning and Identity*. Cambridge: Cambridge University Press.

Wilcock, P. M. (1998). The new NHS: an opportunity for modern, dependable, thinking about quality improvement? *Health Care Quality*, **4**(1–2), 21–5.

Wolcott, H. F. (1988). Ethnographic research in education. In *Complementary Methods for Research in Education* (R. M. Jaeger, ed.) pp. 187–209. Washington, DC: Educational Research Association.

6

Practice knowledge – critical appreciation

Joy Higgs, Della Fish and Rodd Rothwell

INTRODUCTION

Because of continual changes in health and illness phenomena and advances in the related sciences and technologies, practice knowledge in the health fields will continue to face rapid growth as well as rapid obsolescence. Ongoing knowledge generation, testing and refinement are required of professionals. This includes updating, discarding obsolete or unsupported knowledge and expanding knowledge scope and depth. Further, a necessary part of being inducted into professional practice in the first place also requires in learners the ability to appreciate the nature of the practice.

This chapter builds on the arguments presented in Chapter 4, where knowledge and practice were seen as indivisible (as contended by Fish & Coles 1998) and where knowledge discourse was regarded as an attempt to explain practice. In this chapter, we take up this notion of 'attempting to explain' (practice), recognising that the entirety, subtleties and complexities of practice cannot be comprehensively represented within discourses about knowledge. We see knowledge itself as a dynamic phenomenon, changing with developments in practice, and knowledge construction as a way of making sense of our social and physical world that is embedded/situated in our social, cultural, historical and personal contexts. This understanding of practice knowledge is reflected in our deliberate choice of the term 'critical appreciation' in the chapter title to reflect these interpretive frameworks and the notions of challenging and making sense of the complex and changing world of practice.

In this chapter we focus on how, as knowledge generators and users, we employ, create, modify, critically appreciate and validate the wide variety of knowledge we use in practice, by addressing the following questions:

- What do we mean by the use of knowledge in practice and in the appreciation of practice?
- How do concepts of certainty, conviction and truth relate to knowledge construction and appreciation?
- What are the implications for professional practice knowledge of viewing knowledge as a sociohistorically constructed phenomenon that requires critical appreciation?
- How does the context of knowledge construction and use influence its credibility and meaning?
- How are ideas, insights, understandings and experiences of professional practice converted to knowledge?

THE EMPLOYMENT, CREATION AND MODIFICATION OF KNOWLEDGE IN PRACTICE

The activities of a professional practitioner do not involve simply bringing a range of public knowledge (theoretical and practical) into the practice setting and automatically applying this knowledge. For one thing, knowledge generated through research or by theorists, which is inevitably generalised, does not always meet the needs of the particular practice in the field. For another, the knowledge generated by others does not always fit the perceived needs of a particular practitioner who may seek to deconstruct and reconstruct formal theory in terms that make it more intelligible and user-friendly. (This can, of course, involve the misconstruction of the original knowledge!) In Figure 6.1 we identify the different forms of propositional and non-propositional knowledge and the movements (conversions, elaborations, extensions) between the two as they are created, used and modified for and through practice.

It is important for three reasons to consider the practice setting as a vital arena for the construction of new knowledge by practitioners themselves. First, professional judgement is utilised by the professional in the selection of knowledge to be used *and* the kind of use to which that knowledge is put to in the practice setting. Here, the professional considers what is appropriate knowledge, how it might be used and whether it should be modified to suit the particular case. That modification is itself a version of creating knowledge *in* practice. Second, new knowledge may be created in the practice setting, when the professional finds the need to achieve something for which there are no previously developed appropriate procedures, or when the professional meets a version of events which is hitherto unknown or undocumented. Evidence-based practice can exist only in so far as relevant

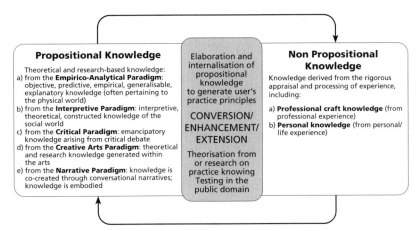

Figure 6.1   Forms of knowledge used in practice and their transformation/enhancement. (From Higgs & Titchen 2000, with permission of Butterworth-Heinemann)

evidence exists and is known about (Ford & Walsh 1994, Grahame-Smith 1995, Beeston & Simons 1996, White 1997, Jones & Higgs 2000)! One thing about which we can be sure, however, in respect of these first two points is that in the practical setting, professionals are continually adapting both formal public and their own informal knowledge to the particular case, or they are extending existing knowledge in response to the current case. Third, and perhaps most significantly, knowledge is created by practitioners in the practice setting by theorising about their practice (that is, by making explicit and refining the tacit knowledge that lies embedded within and beneath the practitioner's actions, activities and know-how).

THE APPRECIATION OF PRACTICE

The activity of appreciating something encompasses notions of 'sensing' and 'becoming aware of', 'understanding' and 'valuing'. In terms of critical appreciation, it is a process in which an activity or an object is examined and understood, by as many means and from as many points of view as possible. This involves considering its creator's or originator's intentions, methods and values, and recognising the traditions and context within which it was created. It means weighing its achievements and failures, seeing in it meanings beyond the surface and recognising that it is representative of a set of principles and beliefs beyond itself. This process can (but need not) lead the 'appreciator' away from the activity or object under review towards larger matters of which it is in some way representative (Fish 2001).

Members of a profession are expected to be able simultaneously to practise and to develop their practice. They utilise discretionary judgement and are self-evaluating (Freidson 1994, 2001). Like all professionals, health science practitioners are required to be their own greatest critics. In relation to their professional knowledge they are expected to be lifelong learners (continually refining and updating their knowledge bases). They are also expected to adopt the stance of a critical self-evaluator who seeks out the best knowledge they have to use (including knowledge they have created in their practice). We expect professionals to recognise when their knowledge is deficient, redundant or irrelevant, and to acknowledge the value of other people's knowledge (including that of their clients) as input to professional decision-making. To achieve these ends it is useful to adopt the model of the connoisseur. Elliot Eisner (1985) conceived of connoisseurship as a form of knowing, describing it as a means of paying attention, accompanied by criticism, being a way of disclosing or expressing what has been seen. Connoisseurs know (*have come to the judgement*) that a painting (for example) is high art, by paying careful attention to all the elements of form and content (and the manner of their interrelation), by considering the painter's intentions and the context of the painting, and by weighing these factors against a developed and developing view of what is 'good', a view that is personal but also resonates with the views of a significant number of others. They are so practised that they make such judgements almost without paying conscious attention to the details of such matters! Eisner argued that in expressing the reasons for their judgements connoisseurs adopt the role of critic, making explicit their knowledge and thus demonstrating how they are linking personal meaning and judgement to more public knowledge. This process of explication expands public knowledge of two kinds (knowledge about the given artefact and knowledge about the bases for such judgements).

Professional practice connoisseurs develop the art and skill of critical appreciation of practice by drawing on both propositional (scientific and theoretical) and procedural (experiential) knowledge of the particular field. They reach an informed judgement which looks beyond technical correctness, efficacy or professional accountability, to examine the more subtle aspects of practice. Just as the connoisseur of fine wine may recognise the subtle delight of an outstanding vintage as well as a poorly produced product, the connoisseur of professional practice can appreciate artistry in practice as well as recognising strengths and deficits in technical expertise. As part of critical appreciation, connoisseurs both develop and contribute to an understanding of key elements that are generally recognised as characterising high quality in professional practice, and they develop a facility in recognising specific versions of those elements. They also learn the skill of reporting on the strengths and limitations of performance and product, by learning and using the language of critique to articulate these attributes. So too, health professionals need language that is relevant to task and audience to articulate their knowledge and their knowledge evaluations.

KNOWLEDGE AS CONSTRUCTION AND CONVICTION

Part of appreciating practice knowledge is asking the questions: What do we mean by knowledge? What counts as true knowledge? Our response is that this is a matter of perspective. As discussed in Chapter 4, people's sociocultural, political context and philosophical perspectives influence what they regard as (true) knowledge.

In this chapter we adopt a constructionist interpretation of knowledge which contends that all knowledge is a construction of human beings who are striving to know about nature and experience. Such knowledge may be constructed by individuals or groups and therefore pertains to the individual's knowledge base or the knowledge of the field. Knowledge in this view arises from a dynamic process of striving to construct or make sense of the world; of taking understandings, insights, observations and experiences and exploring them in relation to existing knowledge, in terms of the perceived realities of experience and other forms of evidence, such as logic and peer review, in order to construct a view of reality that makes sense to the knowledge maker. Numerous methods can be used to generate and explore the validity and usefulness of knowledge, including research, theorising, reasoning, critical debate, reflection on experience, exploration in practice, critical appreciation and argument from first principles.

It is important to specify some contrasts between knowledge understood as construction and knowledge that emerges from the application of experiment. It can be argued that for most of the natural sciences, one method of inquiry dominates. This is referred to as the 'hypothetico-deductive' approach. Hypothetico-deductionism is not so much about the creation or construction of knowledge as we have been discussing above, but about the discovery of empirical 'fact'. This approach does not recognise science as creating knowledge as such, but as finding or discovering what is 'out there in the world/universe', waiting to be discovered. What counts as knowledge here is an account or a theory of what is 'out there'. According to this approach theory is regarded as a representation or a mirror of aspects of the natural world. This is the epistemology of representationalism, the notion that theories (and language) represent nature rather than creating knowledge.

The British philosopher Karl Popper (1959, 1970) was one of the first scholars to articulate this approach as the method of science. In one of the most significant critiques of positivist epistemology (the idea that scientific propositions are given to the senses by nature itself), Popper argued that the discovery of scientific fact begins by a process of theoretical conjecture, not, as the positivists would argue, through objective or empirical observation. This process comprises the elaboration of propositions about the nature of natural phenomena from theoretical constructions, and from these theories comes the deduction of testable hypotheses. Thus, according to Popper, scientists use their creative powers (to produce ideas, even imaginary non-scientific notions) in order to derive conjectures (theories) about natural phenomena. But the hypotheses that are deduced from these theories must be formulated into what Popper calls testable hypotheses. Importantly, by 'testable' Popper means 'falsifiable'. In other words, a scientific hypothesis must be falsifiable through empirical testing and experimentation. Thus empirical tests (or experiments) serve as the criteria for falsifying a theory or hypothesis. For Popper, an unfalsifiable hypothesis (e.g. the proposition that 'it is either raining or not raining in the desert') is not scientific because it cannot be disproved. In epistemological terms, science follows a process or method involving disproof, not proof. The most one can say about one's 'undisproved' hypothesis it that 'so far it has not been disproved'. One cannot speak about truth in the traditional sense, that a hypothesis matches reality precisely or perfectly, but rather that reality has not yet proved the hypothesis incorrect. Thus it is the fact that their theories have withstood the strictures of empirical testing or experimentation that gives scientists a degree of certainty and confidence about them.

The hypothetico-deductive approach, though much debated by many epistemologists, arguably remains the most common epistemological perspective for many of the natural sciences, and also some of the human sciences (especially academic psychology). In short, these scientific communities accept as scientific only those theories (knowledge) that have survived the rigours of testing through observation or experimentation.

It is important to state here that many natural scientists do not regard themselves as following hypothetico-deductive methodology. Some, as indicated in the work of Thomas Kuhn (1970), see themselves as existing within a particular scientific community that specifies, through mutual consensus, its particular method of inquiry. Thus, what will count as knowledge validation (whether it be by observation, testing or experimentation) and even truth is internal to the particular community (or the paradigm, as Kuhn would put it). Some of us are also practising in fields where multiple paradigms occur simultaneously, for example psychology, where different schools of thinking represent different perspectives on what counts as knowledge. This latter perspective allows for diversity in scientific method, in scientific reasoning and in standards of validation, even though we could make the more or less universal statement that empirical testing (whatever it means in practice to the specific community) is the major form of knowledge validation for many of the sciences.

APPRECIATING THE CREDIBILITY OF KNOWLEDGE AS A SOCIOHISTORICAL, POLITICAL CONSTRUCT

In this and other chapters we have discussed the different forms of knowledge or the forms it takes in various contexts and the manner in which it is accepted by a community as relevant and valuable. We argue further here that whatever forms knowledge takes, it does not exist in a vacuum or abstractly, but emerges in a social, cultural and historical context. If we look at all knowledge as being socially conditioned in this contextualised manner, we will come to accept that knowledge serves some useful social or human purpose. It emerges as a means of meeting human needs or solving problems and it is valued for those purposes.

We can see this phenomenon in operation in different cultures. In some societies, for example, the knowledge possessed by priests, shamans and other religious persons is considered crucial for solving serious problems encountered by that community. In agricultural societies, socially sanctioned individuals (shamans, witchdoctors, etc.) may be called upon in times of crisis, such as crop failure in a drought, to use their special knowledge and skills to diagnose what has caused the problem and to indicate how it could be solved. Their advice may also be sought on the curing of physical ills and social and personal conflicts. Often such religious persons are also seen as the mediums who convey important knowledge from spiritual beings. Artists of all varieties are, even in modern industrial society, also perceived as possessing important knowledge that may help people to understand themselves better and to reveal certain truths that are not immediately obvious.

Thus we learn from cultural and historical analysis that we grow up in a social context with already established values about forms of knowledge (and ways of validating that knowledge). Members of a particular society or social group will undergo a process of becoming encultured, which involves learning to internalise these important knowledges. We will internalise a view (or ontology) of the world, its structure, who we are, where we come from, and what is to be valued and not valued. As individuals we will learn how to operate, to cope in our world as members of society. In modern societies this process of individualisation involves becoming a worker, or a person who is identified as having a specific role. There is much to be said about this process that we cannot explore here, but for our purposes we briefly examine the process of becoming a health practitioner, which is in a sense itself a process of individualisation.

We have referred to the process of acquiring knowledge as one of 'internalisation'. We borrow this term from the work of the Russian psychologist and philosopher Vygotsky (1978), who described the process of knowledge/skill acquisition as one of the individual's internalisation of social knowledges and skills. Vygotsky's perspective is that people are constantly developing and changing and that in every situation we have the possibility to gain knowledge from our peers in interactive situations. He described this communal learning situation as the zone of proximal development (ZPD). The ZPD represents the gap between what a person can accomplish individually and what is possible to accomplish under the guidance of adults, mentors or more capable peers (Vygotsky 1978). Vygotsky's (1985) research showed that, through the ZPD, learners operate at a higher level of skill in conjunction with competent peers than they did as individuals without such assistance.

The individual comes into the learning situation as an already encultured person with a background of values, knowledge, skills and understanding. Then a meeting occurs of that background knowledge (etc.) with the new knowledge, skills and values to be learned. According to Vygotsky, the process of learning is one where the learner restructures existing knowledge to incorporate the new knowledge. While in the ZPD, learners are dependent on skilled peers to serve as a knowledge base until they have internalised the knowledge in a manner that enables them to perform new tasks individually without peer assistance.

According to Vygotsky, the process of internalisation is the same as the process of the incorporation of new knowledge. In the ZPD, a person's activities with the help of others involve action and tacit knowledge. With internalisation of that communal activity/tacit knowledge, learners acquire an articulate knowledge of what they are doing and become competent at doing the task without assistance. Vygotsky's view is that action becomes knowledge as it is more or less transmuted into a linguistic form that can be expressed orally or in writing. Learners become independent performers (in a sense, they have internalised the actions of the others in the ZPD) of the particular task. This enables the action to become theorised and opens the possibility for new knowledge to emerge. With this admittedly brief overview of the function of the ZPD we aim to emphasise that the acquisition of knowledge and skills does not occur in a vacuum, but is a communal process that involves a restructuring or reorganisation of individual understanding.

As stated in Chapter 5, learning processes on a personal plane could also be viewed as *participatory appropriation* (Rogoff 1995) to emphasise the dynamic, relational and mutual nature of learning, which is also emphasised in this chapter. This differs from a perspective of learning that refers to pieces of knowledge being transferred from the outside to the inside of the individual. The social and cultural construction of knowledge is discussed further in Chapter 5 (see also Lave & Wenger 1991, Wenger 1998).

New knowledge is confronting. It forces questioning of previous values and entails a new thematic understanding of previously implicit ways of seeing and understanding. It is also an active or dynamic process, where individuals are placed in the position of critics who do not slavishly accept all that their skilled peers say and do and value, but interpret it in the light of their previous and current experience. They may in fact reject the new or emerging knowledge and suggest alternatives. As newcomers to the profession, practitioners have to achieve the competence defined by their professional community to enter the core of its practice, and thus they have to transform their experience until it fits within the regime. This means that they have to learn to view the surrounding world from a certain perspective, to see a situation as, for instance, a physiotherapeutic or a psychological problem.

Thus competence may drive experience. Experience may also drive competence, the perspectives prevailing within a community of practice not being static, but able to be renegotiated and changed. This two-way interaction of experience and competence is, according to Wenger (1998), crucial to the evolution of practice. In it lies the potential for a transformation of both experience and competence and thus for learning, individually and collectively.

It should be pointed out that social circumstances also undergo continuous change. Nothing in a culture remains static. Old values and ways of life and acting become obsolete and are replaced by new ones. This is especially the case in the health field where, for many reasons, new knowledge emerges, new techniques/skills replace old ones, new values in relation to professional activity emerge and social expectations of professional workers change. All these changes impact on professional practice and must be internalised by both new learners and skilled practitioners. While much of this change may well occur around us, it also arises from continuous reflection on our practice.

CREATING KNOWLEDGE FROM IDEAS OF PRACTICE

Since we subscribe to a constructionist view of knowledge and recognise multiple constructions of reality, it would not be reasonable to present here a prescriptive view of how knowledge is created. Indeed, we are focusing on appreciating knowledge, which is an individual (and socially referenced) way of knowing. However, our task here is to explore strategies through which knowledge can come to be appreciated, generated, validated and valued.

In Figure 6.2 we attempt to illustrate a loosely sequenced series of activities which can be included in the process of making sense of the world in order to

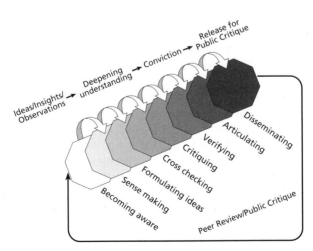

Figure 6.2 Appreciating practice knowledge

produce knowledge. This is not intended to represent an empirical observation or generalisation of knowledge generation in a prescriptive or predictive sense; neither is it a set of rules for generating knowledge. Rather, we propose that a number of interactive, spiralling, reflexive, cognitive and communicative processes and actions can usefully contribute to knowledge development. The sequence commences with the formulation of ideas and proceeds through a deepening understanding of the phenomenon or reality that the thinker is seeking to appreciate. The next phase involves evaluative and critiquing processes which can result in a level of certainty that can be called conviction or validation of the truth (or a sense that the notion is judged to reflect reality satisfactorily). This allows or prompts the knower to release this knowledge claim for public critique. The cycle then progresses through critique by others and by the field, so that knowledge claims become part of the accepted knowledge base of the group/profession/society.

Becoming aware, sense-making and formulating ideas

In their everyday role, health care practitioners are expected to notice things; to become aware of their patients' needs and responses, for instance. But more than this, they are expected to appraise their own performance, role and actions critically. In so doing they can become aware of patterns of behaviour and outcomes in their clinical interventions. For example, they can reflect whether one treatment mode is more effective than another, and under what circumstances. This noticing requires heightened awareness and a learned habit that can be called the development of a 'discerning eye' (Fish 1998). For many practitioners, this awareness may be channelled directly into their clinical role, almost without conscious recognition. That is, they may acquire a large store of mainly tacit knowledge and experience.

Here we face an interesting situation. Tacit knowledge plays an important role in practice. According to Heidegger (1926/1990), craft activity (involving a form of tacit knowledge) must remain tacit to work well. It becomes explicit when the craftspeople make a mistake, such as when sculptors chisel their finger rather than the piece of stone on which they are working. This mistake then focuses the practitioner's consciousness and the activity becomes explicit; the correction is made consciously (or thematically, to use Heidegger's term), by using a better and sharper chisel, for example. Heidegger would argue that craft work must operate on a tacit basis, otherwise it ceases to become craft work and is articulated into a set of guidelines.

In our experience, another way of making tacit knowledge explicit is when practitioners deliberately reflect upon the underlying elements of their practice in order to understand it, communicate it to other practitioners and teach it to students. We would argue that in the context of health care practice, which blends science, art and craft, the wholeness and at times the essence of the artistry or craft of practice cannot be articulated. However, there is much about practice that needs to be further explored and can be made explicit. In particular, experience-based knowledge gained by one practitioner could greatly enhance the practice of others if it is presented to, validated and adopted by the profession. This requires articulation. Thus we make a distinction between, on the one hand, tacit knowledge, which is embedded in the 'do-able' rather than the 'speakable' essence of practice, and on the other, the vast amount of procedural knowledge which awaits exploration, for want either of an explorer or of a tool/mode of exploration. Herein lies much unidentified evidence for practice (but evidence of a different kind from that generated by scientific research).

When we argue, as in this book, that practice epistemology should become part of practice action, as well as the grounding for practice of practitioners as well as researchers, we start with the act of noticing. This awareness does not occur in isolation. Rather, it is embedded in the depth of education and experience of practitioners whose learning, professional socialisation and professional context provide the rich tapestry against which moments of noticing occur. As with the connoisseur who notices a new texture or recognises a repeated theme and then seeks to make sense of this awareness against a tradition of knowledge-making in a discipline, so too the practitioner can pick up a thread of observation or perhaps a persistent idea and examine it against a background of knowing in the practice setting.

In seeking to make sense of a new idea, an insight, an observed pattern or inconsistency, practitioners often explore their existing knowledge base. Does the new idea sit well with what I already know? Is there something unique or new about this situation which means that a new approach is warranted or particularly effective? Does this new knowledge challenge and even invalidate my current 'knowing' (thinking and ideas)? How can I connect my findings or activities across a number of cases to derive some sense of what appears to be happening in my practice? Is there a human variable (e.g. the patient's choice or interests) which makes me recognise that some different technique or rationale is necessary here? Self-questioning and reflection play a major role here in appreciating the subtleties of a situation and developing understandings and explanations.

In reflecting on their practice, health professionals could take a philosophical approach through which they endeavour to understand the essence and meaning of their practice and its settings. A particular challenge could be to frame ontological questions, that is, questions concerned with knowing in being, with how the knower views the world and with how one's view of the world influences how one creates and uses knowledge. Alternatively, epistemological questions could be framed, that is, questions about the nature of knowledge itself, that ask how people make sense of their world.

Cross-checking and critiquing

Health professionals frequently try out new ideas, variations, techniques and strategies in practice. This active experimentation within practice is part of both creating new knowledge and cross-checking emerging knowledge. Similarly, this checking may take the form of self-debate. The new idea or potential intervention strategy can be analysed, deconstructed, examined from multiple perspectives to further the process of refining and testing it out. Questions form part of this process: Why should this (pattern, idea, understanding) be so? Does it make sense? What is confusing me about this knowledge/idea? How can I sort out these confusions or inconsistencies? Can I apply this knowledge in my practice? The issue of the compatibility of new knowledge with the knowledge base of an individual is a critical factor in clinical effectiveness. In clinical reasoning the practitioner often needs to deal with and make sense of differences between new knowledge and existing propositional and experience-based knowledge. Conflicts between such forms of knowledge could be due to the presence of existing knowledge that is obsolete, inadequate, incomplete, erroneous or irrelevant to the given situation, or there could be a problem with the new knowledge. Or there could, in this complex and subtle world in which we live, be ideas about some aspect of health care which remain irreconcilable, and the practitioner needs to be able to make professional judgements to deal with this situation.

In reflecting and deliberating on practice the professional has many questions to address. How well is this knowledge/procedure working in my practice? Why does this treatment or argument work? If I try to explain it (e.g. action, finding, notion) based on my propositional knowledge, can I find a satisfactory explanation? (For example, can my knowledge of biomechanics, anatomy or physiology help to explain why an invented treatment technique or variation should work?) What could be the possible consequences of taking this course of action? How does this new approach sit with the professional knowledge base and the literature pertaining to evidence-based practice? In using this knowledge or technique in my practice, does my self-knowledge and my knowledge of ethics, culture and professional standards create ease of use or difficulties?

Interestingly, we are raising a number of questions about the questions being explored. Not only are we seeking to find some truth (or matching with reality) but also some rightness, justification and compatibility with self and others in the use of this knowledge in practice. To critique, then, includes dealing with issues of relevance and appropriateness for the setting (e.g. individual client, culture, professional role).

Verifying

Verification of claims to knowledge requires rigour and conviction. Rigour in knowledge generation is both an intention (to seek truth) and an approach (including providing transparency of method to facilitate critique, being systematic and thorough to test truth with open-mindedness in the pursuit of clarity and truthfulness). Yet the nature of the rigour is also dependent upon the knowledge tradition being utilised. In the positivist tradition, the requirement for rigour arises from the goal of the research to generalise from its findings. Here rigour is manifest in strict adherence to rules of the scientific method (e.g. objectivity, reliability and validity) and to the protocols of experimental research (e.g. random allocation of subjects, blind trials, statistical significance).

In keeping with the aim of the professional artist to generate meaning rather than to develop propositional knowledge, the major instrument for collection of evidence in the connoisseurship model is the practitioner through whom the meaning is developed and expressed (Eisner 1981). Eisner also emphasised the importance of the connoisseur as a way of communicating meaning in a manner that is understandable to the relevant community. If no one but the connoisseur can recognise the description, it will not be regarded as a competent interpretation. Rigour associated with the expertise of critical appreciation (the processes, language and form) develops within the context of a critical community, as argued by Schön (1983), who proposed that the professional knowledge by which practitioners 'make sense of practice situations, formulate goals and directions for action, and determine what constitutes acceptable professional conduct' is 'embedded within the socially and institutionally constructed context shared by a community of practitioners' (p. 33).

Rigour associated with professional artistry must include rigour within both the development and the expression of artistry, if the relevant professional community is to adopt the artistic evidence before them. Rigour to achieve artistry is not only a planned cognitive activity as a component of systematic reflection-on-action for instance, but also requires the application of a high level of awareness or attention to thinking within practice (Beeston & Higgs 2001, p. 114).

Beyond individual critique and metacognitive scrutiny, rigour is achieved by peer critique through validating knowledge by exposing it to the professional community (as discussed below).

Conviction is a decision and a judgement rather than a point of absolute certainty. To be convinced that a claim to knowledge has been verified, knowers need to have reached a point where they believe that the evidence accumulated is sufficient to judge the claim to be acceptable or true. Ayer (1956, p. 222) argued that when seeking to verify knowledge claims we should take scepticism of these claims seriously, since it will enable us to learn 'to distinguish the different levels at which our claims to knowledge stand'. Thus, knowing is a continual process of generating, refining and understanding knowledge. In Chapter 4 the various ways that knowledge can be classified were explored, and each form of knowledge, it was argued, can be used as evidence for both conducting and exploring practice.

Articulating

One of the most difficult challenges in knowledge generation is to articulate knowledge clearly, sensibly and in a form and language meaningful to the knowledge-using community. In a health profession, that community is likely to include professional practitioners and their clients, so that different (properly appropriate) forms of expression are required to take account of different medical knowledge and different linguistic backgrounds.

Articulation (oral and written) of new practice knowledge may take the form of definitions, explanations, illustrations, examples and arguments. The role of writing in enabling practitioners to clarify, sharpen and share their new understandings is vital. This is not merely about writing as a finished product. Writing is itself a creative process that facilitates the creation of new knowledge. It facilitates the reshaping of the writer's thinking, and the sharing of drafts with others. Thus, before publication, writing provides the means to engage in and draw upon the collective wisdom of the practitioner's immediate community, while after publication it engenders further discussion and debate. The struggle with writing drafts is itself a struggle with meaning, as well as with clarifying the means of communicating that meaning. Meaning emerges from the writing just as an artefact emerges from the work of the artist; and it often surprises the artist or writer. The process of writing (or making meaning) takes the originator beyond what was planned and what was known at the beginning. Writing enables writers to discover what they really think, understand and want to say. And it is precisely because the evolution of new knowledge emerges through a series of drafts, which seek to capture complex ideas in order to refine them, that the oral tradition does not provide a sufficient basis for developing professional practice (Fish 1998).

Disseminating and peer reviewing

Practice knowledge varies across different health professions and within individual professions as they work with specific client groups or within specific contexts of care (Beeston & Higgs 2001). In this way knowledge and practice norms and traditions are social entities which emerge from practice and are shared by communities of practitioners. According to Krefting (1991), the rigour of peer review by professional communities is concerned with credibility and transferability rather than with validity. In relation to the practice knowledge inherent in professional artistry, the credibility of this knowledge 'requires that others in the community of practice find the meaning that is expressed to be credible in terms of the traditions of practice, and that they find it can be transferred to their own practice and applied in other contexts' (Beeston & Higgs 2001, p. 114).

Dissemination of knowledge in professional communities occurs via conference presentations, journal articles and other publications, educational programmes and informal communications. As part of presenting the new knowledge to the field to allow for wider consideration and investigation, articulation of the knowledge should also include description of how it was generated and in what context, so that the knowledge claim can be critiqued.

Ongoing development

Ongoing development of knowledge is part of the search for truth in a changing world. Despite the importance of knowledge validation, it is essential also to see knowledge as a developing or dynamic phenomenon. Kleinig (1982, p. 152), for instance, argued that 'the knowing subject must continually reflect on and test what [knowledge] is presented'. Practitioners need to develop an appreciation of the credibility of their knowledge; to be able to defend their knowledge, but at the same time to acknowledge that much of the range and depth of their knowledge has conditional certainty in terms of contextual relevance and durability.

Therefore, knowledge claims developed by individuals or groups need to be critiqued and validated in the field in practice settings. At one level, such validation would appear to be a simple matter; it is concerned with whether the knowledge actually 'works' in practice. But seeing what works is often not a simple matter of measuring a patient outcome on a single occasion. The improvement in the patient may be subtle and visible only over time. Certainly this may be evaluated by empirical means. However, another important element of the validation of the new knowledge in the practice setting involves a critical appreciation of the professional practice within which the new knowledge is being activated. Appreciating such practice is a matter of developing the discerning eye of the connoisseur, and taking a holistic view of the piece of practice. It entails not rushing to a quick critique, but rather 'allowing the ... [new] practice to make its impact and reporting what it was that made that impact' and what made it valuable (Fish 1998, p. 197). Appreciating practice involves:

- understanding the context (the history, traditions and physical context) within which the practice is carried out
- discerning beneath professional practice the professional's aims, intentions and, above all, vision
- being clear about the moral ends of the practice and the appropriateness of the means to these ends
- being aware of the worth of the practice as professional practice
- recognising the professional's skills, capacities and abilities, theories, values, emotions, beliefs and personal qualities
- seeing the artistic nature of the performance and perceiving what the professional has done to achieve this artistry
- discerning within practice the fusion (the balance and harmony, integration and unity) of the visible with the invisible (skills, thoughts,

theories, values, abilities, emotions and personal qualities), and thus discerning the value of the practice as a whole
- identifying the employment of imagination within the practice
- distinguishing and distilling out from this picture the observer's own vision (Fish 1998, pp. 205–206).

For practitioners, then, the understanding and development of practice is not a matter of looking at practice via theory, but of working from within practice itself to enquire into practice (Eraut 1994, Fish 1998, Fish & Coles 1998). This will allow us to refine new knowledge and its use, and to identify areas where still further knowledge is needed. It may also lead us to discover new visions of what is involved in professional practice itself.

However, we should recognise that there is much about practice which is unknown and difficult to articulate (Polanyi 1966). This quality has been described by Eraut (1994, p. 15): 'Critics may illuminate the knowledge embedded in a piece of music, a painting or a dance, but they cannot fully represent it in words'.

In addition to the generation of knowledge in practice, research about practice is a vital way of exploring practice knowledge. Beyond the individual's role in developing professional craft knowledge is the contribution that this knowledge can make to the knowledge base of the profession. The initial part of this process requires research that identifies the professional craft knowledge of experienced practitioners with regard to particular problems and contexts through insider practitioner research (Fish 1998, Higgs et al 2001). After the identification of dimensions of practice, particularly of expert practice, empirical research may then be used to test the efficacy of that knowledge more broadly across a range of practitioners and settings. Through this testing process, the professional craft knowledge of individuals is transformed into propositional knowledge of the profession. It is then ready to be reconsidered by practitioners themselves. And so the endless spiral of the development and use of knowledge in professional practice continues.

REFERENCES

Ayer, A. J. (1956). *The Problem of Knowledge*. London: Penguin Books.
Beeston, S. & Higgs, J. (2001). Professional practice: artistry and connoisseurship. In *Practice Knowledge and Expertise in the Health Professions* (J. Higgs & A. Titchen, eds) pp. 108–17. Oxford: Butterworth-Heinemann.
Beeston, S. & Simons, H. (1996). Physiotherapy practice: practitioners' perspectives. *Physiotherapy Theory and Practice*, **12**, 231–42.
Eisner, E. (1981). On the differences between scientific and artistic approaches to qualitative research. *Educational Reader*, April, pp. 5–9.
Eisner, E. W. (1985). *The Art of Educational Evaluation: A Personal View*. London: Falmer Press.
Eraut, M. (1994). *Developing Professional Knowledge and Competence*. London: Falmer Press.
Fish, D. (1998). *Appreciating Practice in the Caring Professions: Refocusing Professional Development and Practitioner Research*. Oxford: Butterworth-Heinemann.

Fish, D. (2001). Mentoring and the artistry of professional practice. In *Mentoring in the New Millennium: A Selection of Papers from the Second British Council Regional Mentor Conference*, pp. 11–26. Cluj-Napocca, Romania: Editura Napocca Star.

Fish, D. & Coles, C. (eds) (1998). *Developing Professional Judgement in Health Care: Learning Through the Critical Appreciation of Practice*. Oxford: Butterworth-Heinemann.

Ford, P. & Walsh, M. (1994). *New Rituals for Old: Nursing Through the Looking Glass*. Oxford: Butterworth-Heinemann.

Freidson, E. (1994). *Professionalism Reborn: Theory, Prophesy and Policy*. Cambridge: Polity Press.

Freidson, E. (2001). *Professionalism: The Third Logic*. Cambridge: Polity Press.

Grahame-Smith, D. (1995). Evidence-based medicine: Socratic dissent. *British Medical Journal*, **310**, 1126–7.

Heidegger, M. (1926/1990). *Being and Time*. Oxford: Basil Blackwell. (Translated from the German *Sein und Zeit* by John Macquarrie and Edward Robinson.)

Higgs, J. (2001). Charting standpoints in qualitative research. In *Critical Moments in Qualitative Research* (H. Byrne-Armstrong, J. Higgs & D. Horsfall, eds) pp. 44–67. Oxford: Butterworth-Heinemann.

Higgs, J. & Titchen, A. (2000). Knowledge and reasoning. In *Clinical Reasoning in the Health Professions*, 2nd edn (J. Higgs & M. Jones, eds) pp. 23–32. Oxford: Butterworth-Heinemann.

Higgs, J. Titchen, A. & Neville, V. (2001). Professional practice and knowledge. In *Practice Knowledge and Expertise in the Health Professions* (J. Higgs & A. Titchen, eds) pp. 3–9. Oxford: Butterworth-Heinemann.

Jones, M. & Higgs, J. (2000). Will evidence-based practice take the reasoning out of practice? In *Clinical Reasoning in the Health Professions*, 2nd edn (J. Higgs & M. Jones, eds) pp. 307–15. Oxford: Butterworth-Heinemann.

Kleinig, J. (1982). *Philosophical Issues in Education*. London: Routledge.

Krefting, L. (1991). The culture concept in the everyday practice of occupational and physical therapy. *Physical and Occupational Therapy in Pediatrics*, **11**(4), 1–16.

Kuhn, T. S. (1970). *The Structure of Scientific Revolutions*, 2nd edn. Chicago: University of Chicago Press.

Lave, J. & Wenger, E. (1991). *Situated Learning: Legitimate Peripheral Participation*. Cambridge, MA: Cambridge University Press.

Polanyi, M. (1966). *The Tacit Dimension*. Garden City, NY: Doubleday.

Popper, K. (1959). *The Logic of Scientific Discovery*. Cambridge: Cambridge University Press.

Popper, K. R. (1970). Normal science and its dangers. In *Criticism and the Growth of Knowledge* (I. Lakatos & A. Musgrave, eds) pp. 51–58. New York: Cambridge University Press.

Rogoff, B. (1995). Observing socio-cultural activity on three planes: participatory appreciation, guided participation, and apprenticeship. In *Socio-Cultural Studies of Mind* (J. V. Wertsch, ed.) pp. 139–64. Cambridge: Cambridge University Press.

Schön, D. (1983). *The Reflective Practitioner: How Professionals Think in Action*. New York: Basic Books.

Vygotsky, L. S. (1978). *Mind in Society: The Development of Higher Psychological Process*. Cambridge, MA: Harvard University Press.

Vygotsky, L. S. (1985). *Thought and Language*, transl. A. Kozulin. Cambridge, MA: MIT Press.

Wenger, E. (1998). *Communities of Practice: Learning, Meaning and Identity*. Cambridge: Cambridge University Press.

White, S. (1997). Evidence-based practice and nursing: the new panacea? *British Journal of Nursing*, **6**, 175–8.

7

Blending self-knowledge and professional knowledge in person-centred care

Angie Titchen and Maeve McGinley
(with Brendan McCormack)

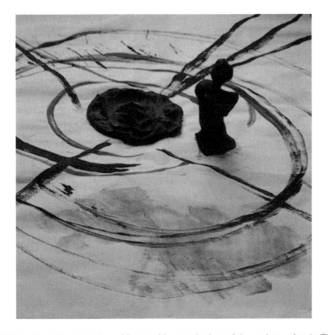

(The painting above is reproduced here with permission of the painter, Angie Titchen.)

In the pasture of this world, I endlessly push aside the tall grasses in search of the bull.
Following unnamed rivers, lost upon the interpenetrating paths of distant mountains.
My strength failing and my vitality exhausted, I cannot find the bull.
I only hear the locusts chirring through the forest at night ...
(The verses quoted in this chapter are from *Zen Flesh, Zen Bones*, compiled by Paul Reps (1957).)

Expertise in person-centred health care requires the professional to use and blend different knowledges and diverse ways of knowing and being. Such expertise involves the blending of self-knowledge and intellectual, emotional and personal maturity with the person's professional knowledge base. This knowledge base is formed by: (1) propositional or theoretical knowledge derived through research and scholarship; (2) professional craft knowledge acquired through professional experience; and (3) personal knowledge accrued through life experience (Higgs & Titchen 2000; Fig. 7.1). Systematic critique enables the development of each kind of knowledge. The blending of these knowledges appears to enable the therapeutic use of self within the practitioner–patient relationship. However, these knowledges are often tacit and deeply embedded in the practitioner, and in the practice itself, which makes it difficult to establish if and how they are blended. The limited amount of research in this field suggests that such blending requires critical review and control of one's knowledge base (Eraut 1994, Titchen 2000, RCN 2002). This research also shows that we need an understanding of how the different knowledges in this base are created, verified and blended, and an evaluation of their usefulness in decision-making in particular situations.

Along the riverbank under the trees, I discover footprints!
Even under the fragrant grass I see his prints.
Deep in remote mountains they are found.
These traces no more can be hidden than one's nose, looking heavenward.

Until recently, this blending was largely ignored and undervalued by the practitioners who were clearly doing it, but in barely conscious and unreflective ways. It was ignored and unvalued also in research and education, with researchers and educators being mostly concerned with the creation, application and learning of propositional knowledge, in ways often far removed from practice itself. So the processes of generating knowledge in and from practice, by practitioners, and its blending with other forms of knowledge appeared somewhat mysterious and ineffable when people in the health sciences began to take more interest in these tasks.

This chapter is a walk through the search for the knowledges inherent in person-centred care and their blending. Just as the ancient wisdom of Zen and Celtic stories show meandering and fruitless searches for the bull, the holy grail or whatever, we demonstrate that the knowledge that we are searching for does not lie somewhere 'out there', rather it lies 'within'.

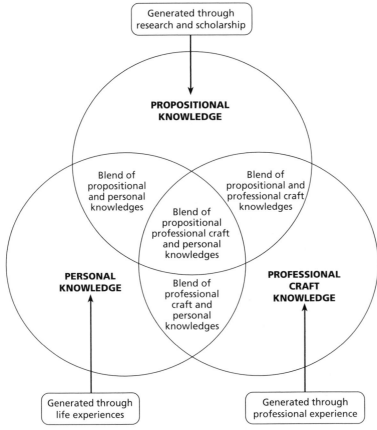

Figure 7.1   Forms and derivation of knowledge. (After Higgs & Titchen 2000, with permission of Butterworth-Heinemann.)

We enter the mystery of practice 'within' by using vignettes of therapeutic use of self in professional practice and reflecting on its impact on patients. The vignettes arise from two action research studies in which we have taken part (Binnie & Titchen 1999, RCN 2002). Using metaphor and critical dialogue, we examine the nature of the therapeutic use of self in a nurse (Maeve McGinley) with expertise in working with people who have bladder and bowel problems. We explore her knowledge and her ways of knowing and being. We contrast the way she uses herself therapeutically in practice with others.

Barefooted and naked of breast, I mingle with the people of the world.
My clothes are ragged and dust-laden, and I am ever blissful.
I use no magic to extend my life;
Now, before me, the dead trees become alive.

Through this exploration of two key aspects of health and social care – first, the way the professional's role is enhanced by a therapeutic use of self, and second, how different knowledges are used by the practitioner to optimise person-centred care – we seek answers to the important question, 'How can understanding the nature and generation of knowledge facilitate a person-centred approach to health and social care?' (We use these two latter terms to be inclusive of different modes/settings of practice, including regular health settings and other non-health settings, e.g. schools, workplaces, community venues, where health professionals work in health and social service roles.) We look first 'within', at specifics, and then move out towards generalities. Moreover, by critically dialoguing with practice, we show how the knowledges of practice can be generated and tested, in practice, through reflection, using research-based analytical tools and critical dialogue. And, rather like unpacking a set of Russian dolls, we discover that the facilitator of reflection and dialogue uses similar strategies and values to those used by practitioners giving person-centred care.

INTRODUCTION

Person-centredness rests in the ethics of care. Increasingly, clinically effective care is being seen as both evidence-based and person-centred. This means that the right treatment, given in the right way, for the right patient, at the right time, is delivered in ways that address the needs and concerns of the particular patient as he or she sees them. Both evidence-based and person-centred care draw on holistic practice knowledges. Professionals, therefore, need to be aware of their own practice knowledge base, which includes their personal knowledge and knowing how they put their values into action.

Health care researchers often look for these knowledges on the mountain tops, seeking an objective reality and ignoring the values of individuals. However, the research approaches they use may result in skeletal lists of decontextualised essences and abstractions (Parse et al 1985, Forrest 1989) of professional practice that is essentially complex, unique, subjective and value-laden. Increasingly researchers, and especially practitioner–researchers such as ourselves, have abandoned the search on the mountain tops, the search for the bull. Instead, we seek these knowledges and values, and the ways they are used in practice, by looking within ourselves, our contexts and situations, celebrating and explicating the unique and subjective. By using a range of theoretical tools and perspectives, this work can then be transformed to become potentially transferable to other settings, people and contexts (Titchen & Ersser 2001).

In this chapter we use analytical tools developed through empirical or scholarly research by Manley and McCormack (1997), Higgs and Titchen (2000), Titchen and Higgs (2001) and Titchen (2001a, 2001b) and put them to work with evidence from Maeve's portfolio of evidence which she compiled for recognition of her expertise in her specialty (RCN 2002). Through this process, we render Maeve's subjective experience potentially transferable to other health care professionals in other fields of practice. Whether we achieve this aim rests on your judgement of the usefulness of our contextualised, theoretical principles in your setting. (Please note that we use the terms 'patient' and 'carer' because this is what Maeve calls those with whom she works. Where we are theorising, the term should be taken to include the terms that you use to refer to those with whom you work in partnership, such as, 'client', 'school child' or 'community'.)

Maeve investigated her own practice in the Royal College of Nursing's Expertise in Practice Project with the help of her critical companion, Brendan McCormack. A critical companion is an experienced facilitator (often, but not necessarily, a colleague) who accompanies a practitioner on an experiential learning journey towards person-centred care. This outcome is sought by helping practitioners to become more aware of first, how they bring the self as a human being into the relationship with the patient/client, and second, the nature of their professional knowledge base that informs their practice, and how it was generated. The first area can be thought of as the ontology of practice (cf. Freshwater 1998, Higgs & Titchen 2001), referring to our ways of being (e.g. being sensitive or authentic in our relationships). The second area can be conceptualised as the epistemology of practice, or what we know, how we know it and how we create knowledge. Maeve's increased awareness of her ontology and epistemology of practice opened up the possibility of scrutiny, with Brendan, of her ways of being and knowing in practice. This awareness has also helped her to create knowledge, both in and from her own practice.

Maeve and Brendan used a variety of methods and data sources to gather robust, verifiable evidence for critical scrutiny. Methods included Maeve's critical reflections on the care of her patients, 360° feedback from her role-set (colleagues who would give her honest, challenging, constructive and detailed feedback about her care), and a user narrative by someone receiving Maeve's care. We present some of that evidence here, as a story, to show Maeve's ways of being human and acting out her values and her holistic practice knowledge. The story also demonstrates her journey towards becoming a critical companion to her colleagues. We engage in a critical dialogue with the story. To differentiate between dialogue and story, we use a different typeface for the latter.

MAEVE'S BLENDING OF DIFFERENT KNOWLEDGES TO OPTIMISE PERSON-CENTRED CARE

The scene is set by Maeve's (M) summary reflection on reading her user's narrative. The user, Kate, is the mother and carer of Maeve's patient, Joseph, an 18-year-old boy with an undiagnosed neurodegenerative condition. (Kate,

Joseph and Sean (Kate's husband) are pseudonyms.) Kate was interviewed by Brendan, who analysed the narrative using the attributes of expertise (Manley & McCormack 1997). These attributes are *holistic practice knowledge, knowing the patient, saliency, moral agency* and *skilled know-how*. We hear from Kate (K) and Brendan (B) later.

> *M:* I feel that this narrative is a very powerful piece. It reflects enormous trust in me by Kate to so willingly share her story with Brendan. The narrative would appear to clearly indicate that as a clinical practitioner I demonstrate all the attributes of expertise and I am an effective skilled companion for the carers, patient and others involved in this case.
>
> Illustrated in this narrative is when and how I demonstrate the various attributes and also some outcomes. For example, Kate talked about how until I came along no one seemed to know why her son had so many infections, but I was able to identify that he might have incomplete bladder emptying which could be the cause. Brendan identified from what Kate said that I knew what was the appropriate course of action to take and I applied a variety of knowledge to the situation in order to make the most appropriate decisions (technical and aesthetic). This he took to be a demonstration of skilled know-how and he highlighted the outcome in that the patient received appropriate treatment to prevent any further infections and Kate felt relieved and thankful.
>
> Using Titchen's (2001a) 'skilled companionship' model [Fig. 7.2] to analyse my expertise within this narrative, I sensed that I clearly demonstrated expertise as a skilled

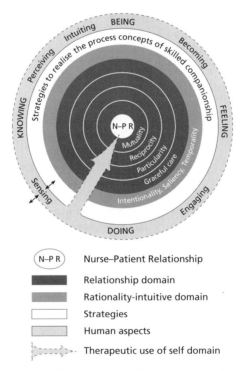

N-P R — Nurse–Patient Relationship

Relationship domain

Rationality-intuitive domain

Strategies

Human aspects

Therapeutic use of self domain

Figure 7.2 Skilled companionship: a conceptual framework for person-centred health care. (From Titchen 2000, with permission of Ashdale Press.)

companion to Joseph and his carers. My domains (relationship, rationality–intuitive, therapeutic use of self) appeared to be strong and very well-balanced. I seemed to manage, effectively, the fine interplay between my intuitive and rational judgment and between my theoretical and professional craft knowledge. The practical strategies that I had adopted to realise the process concepts, within the domains, appeared to have been effective. For example, within the narrative it is highlighted how I was able to identify the key risk factors for the patient through using my holistic knowledge (*saliency*) and how I would speak to doctors on Kate's behalf because I sensed she felt uncomfortable contacting them, as she felt they did not always listen to her (*particularity*). How I demonstrate *graceful care* with this patient appeared to be illustrated when Kate said, *'I feel comfortable with Maeve being in the house, I don't feel I have to put on a show for her, you know, and she knows all the different things that are going on. Maybe it's just Maeve herself, the person that she is, she just makes it easy to relax with her'.* An example of the therapeutic use of self domain being illustrated by me was when Kate said, *'Maeve really listens to everything you say, and I find, like the hospital appointments, you know you're slotted into a certain time and I understand that, but I don't believe they listen to you. Maeve listens to everything you say and she thinks about it and she'd maybe come up with a few suggestions, but she leaves it open, you know, she leaves a lot open to us to decide ...'.*

... The content of this narrative is both humbling and reassuring that I have been effective in achieving what I want to be, an expert skilled companion to my patient and his carers.

In this excerpt we can see Maeve drawing on different kinds of knowledge and, beneath that, her valuing of person-centred care. Her role-set also talked about her 'in depth knowledge – not in books', using 'experiential' knowledge, drawing 'from theoretical knowledge and working knowledge', being 'hands on when addressing a problem', 'no gaps/seamless knowledge' and 'knows theory and relates it in a practical sense'. Also evident were her values in action, for example, being 'patient-centred', having an 'attitude of caring' and a 'genuine concern for patients'.

Three types of knowledge (Fig. 7.1) are clear in Maeve's evidence. They appear seamless in her practice. She uses them simultaneously, as represented by the overlap of the three circles. She shapes or influences her theoretical (propositional) knowledge, her working knowledge (professional craft knowledge) and her attitudes and concern (personal knowledge – awareness of her values), each with the other, as represented by the circles where they overlap. By shaping or influencing, we mean that each type of knowledge imbues the other, thus changing it in some way. We discuss this transformation later.

In this excerpt, we also see that Maeve wants affirmation that skilled companionship (Fig. 7.2) is evident in her practice. Skilled companionship is a conceptual framework derived from a phenomenological case study of patient-centred nursing. The framework is supported by empirical research literature (Titchen 2000) and in practice development work in a variety of health care professional fields (e.g. RCN 2002). The framework describes three practical knowledge domains, the know-how of person-centred health care.

In the investigation of her own practice, Maeve finds strong and balanced evidence of all three domains. This balance and the interplay she mentions between the domains and between rational thinking and intuition, all within the therapeutic use of self-domain, constitute what Titchen calls professional artistry. We return to this artistry notion later when we consider the transformation of knowledge, its use and creation. For now, we focus on some of the skilled companionship know-how in action.

Maeve refers to *saliency*, which means the ability to know both consciously and intuitively what is important and needs to be attended to, both from the practitioner's and the patient's/carer's perspectives. Practitioners focus on significant cues and clues, planning care that will address what matters both to them and to patients/carers. Maeve also refers to *particularity*, which means getting to know and understand the unique details of a patient/carer as a person, within both the context of the specific illness situation and the context of the person's life. In addition, Maeve points out *graceful care*, which refers to using all aspects of self in an authentic way, using our bodies, comportment and humour, bringing our spirituality, appropriate emotions and engagement into care, being generous and offering unconditional love. Within graceful caring, more than anywhere else, we see a practitioner's way of being (ontology) in action. Listen to Kate's experience of graceful care:

> K: Maeve's just so easy to talk to and I mean Maeve would keep saying, 'Just ring me any time at work'. I would be a bit reluctant to ring [just] anybody. I feel happier, if I was going to have to ring anybody, Maeve would be the first person I would go to.
>
> B: Really. Why's that?
>
> K: Because she just makes herself so available you know, she makes you feel comfortable that, if you ring her, you don't feel like you're bothering her, and she's so busy and I'm aware that she is busy but she never gives that impression, she always gives you the impression that she's plenty of time for you, you know, she'll come in and see you.
>
> B: Yes. So did that make you feel cared for at the time?
>
> K: Yes, definitely …
> … Maeve's more like a friend now. We would just think Maeve's a friend rather than a nurse. I find her easier to talk to than anybody else that's coming in, plus the fact because she has seen Joseph in so many different sort of situations and moods and different things, she sees the picture, and Maeve just seems to be able to pick up on things. It's unbelievable you know. She understands better than anybody …
> … She's genuinely interested in what is going on here. She is concerned about Joseph as a person and she's concerned about us as his family.

Brendan's analytic commentary on this evidence follows:

> B: Throughout the interview, Kate spoke of Maeve like a 'family friend' and indeed in discussion with Maeve, she spoke of the family like her friends also. Maeve is the first point of contact for Kate and clearly she relies on Maeve to clear a path through the complexities of the health and social care system that she has to cope with. Maeve is clearly a skilled companion to Kate. She spoke passionately about Maeve's caring

approach to Joseph, her care about her [Kate] as a carer and care about the whole situation …

… Many theorists have identified 'being a friend' as a component of the therapeutic caring relationship (e.g. Boykin & Schoenhofer 1993). Here Kate talks freely of the importance of Maeve's friendship. Maeve has broken the boundaries that often exist in a professional caring relationship ('we would just think Maeve's a friend rather than a nurse'). She sees the whole picture and works with Joseph and his mother to make appropriate decisions.

This last sentence shows *saliency* and *mutuality* in action. Mutuality means working with, rather than doing to, and describes the working together of the professional, the patient and the family in a genuine partnership. Professionals offer their expertise as a resource to maximise patients' and families' control in their own care and recovery, and to help them deal with the consequences of illness and find their own solutions. For example, Maeve's knowledge of the health care system enables Kate and her husband to make a variety of decisions and to plan their consultations with the doctors to gain as much as they can from the experience.

> *K:* I spoke to Maeve on the phone and she was more or less sort of saying to me, sit down and write down the things you want to ask and think about it, and go through a few of the things that we have been talking about. So that did help me because I did that.

Kate experiences mutuality as linked with Maeve's extensive knowledge base and as beneficial for her:

> *K:* Maeve listens to everything you say and she thinks about it and she'd maybe come up with a few suggestions but she leaves it open, you know, she leaves a lot open to us to decide …

Brendan points out:

> *B:* Of all the qualities that Maeve possesses and that are valued by Kate, her ability to listen is the one she appreciates most. This is a constant theme throughout the narrative – Maeve listens and thus gets to know the family and makes appropriate decisions that are 'family-centred' because of her ability to hear what the family are saying and thus recognise how best to help them.

> *K:* Maeve respects what you say, she makes it easier you know, but if Maeve suggests something, I will listen and I'll think about it, because of who she is, because of the way she behaves, because, as I said, Maeve is like a friend and everybody feels the same about her. With a friend, you respect friends, so you'll listen to a friend, I'm not saying you don't listen to the district nurses, but … they're just doing the dressing, asking how he is … and away again … Maeve realises how difficult it is and understands and she's very sympathetic. She doesn't start criticising anything we do, even maybe if it's not what she agrees with, she never criticises you or anything or makes you feel that you're doing it wrong.

Kate experiences both Maeve's bringing herself as a person into her care (personal and professional craft knowledges) and her technical expertise (propositional knowledge) as therapeutic:

> *K:* Because Maeve's coming into the house, she sees everything that's going on. I mean, we've other children in the house. I feel comfortable with Maeve being in the house, I don't

feel I have to put on a show for her you know, and she knows all the different things that are going on. Maybe it's just Maeve herself, the person that she is, she just makes it easy to relax with her. She's very knowledgeable, so if Joseph does have a problem, I find that the fact you have Maeve here, you've a better chance of finding out exactly what's wrong, even if you go to the doctor you know, and then she can liaise with the doctor.

So where is this story leading? Together with an increasing amount of research evidence (Brown 1986, Bottorff 1991, Taylor 1992, Ersser 1997, Binnie & Titchen 1999, Edwards 2002), the story demonstrates that using a wealth of technical, propositional knowledge is not enough for some patients and families. They also want professionals who know how to offer a partnership, who value patients'/carers' knowledge and facilitate their involvement in care and decision-making. They want professionals who know how to offer their propositional and professional craft knowledges as a resource and how to tailor this knowledge to help their particular situation and illness experience. They want professionals who know how to make themselves approachable and 'more like a friend'. Thus some patients want the practitioner's technical knowledge, practical know-how and personal knowledge used in practice, and they want them used in a seamless way. This evidence from patients/clients and their families also suggests that they experience the professional role as being enhanced by the therapeutic use of self. There is an increasing amount of evidence that professionals, like Maeve, also experience an enhancement of the professional role in this way (Benner 1984, McMahon & Pearson 1991, Ersser 1997, Binnie & Titchen 1999).

The story and critical dialogue, so far, have indicated how different knowledges are used by practitioners to optimise evidence-based, person-centred care. In the next section we attempt to strengthen the link between the blending of types of knowledge and the outcome of person-centred care, by examining how practitioners with less insight into the nature of their professional practice knowledge base (and how they develop and refine it) fail to optimise person-centred care to its fullest extent, despite well-developed personal and interpersonal skills, the very stuff (one might think) of person-centred care.

LESS THAN OPTIMAL CARE

In her portfolio, Maeve reflected on why colleagues with whom she had worked in the past saw Maeve as possessing a vastly greater and almost unattainable repertoire of knowledge than themselves. Maeve's involvement in the Expertise in Practice project had made her conscious of the nature of her knowledge base and helped her to become increasingly analytical of the knowledges that she was using and how she was blending and balancing them. This new consciousness led her to examine her former colleagues' knowledge bases, using the skilled companionship framework:

> *M:* I see that while my colleagues' relationship domain (how they relate to patients in practice) is particularly good, I can also see that in terms of the other domains, particularly the rationality–intuitive domain, they are weak … Their weakness is evident when they are discussing cases with which they are having a problem and sometimes when they are communicating with GPs about patients and are asked to justify their thinking. Whenever we discuss problem cases, I can see that I pull out the salient points of the case quickly, but they, more often, cannot. Also I will tend, in these cases, to identify investigations and additional information that they would need in order to get to the bottom of the problem … If I challenge their knowledge and reasoning, such as why they selected a particular treatment, they often cannot articulate their underpinning knowledge or give supporting arguments or provide evidence to support their decision to select the treatment offered. I, in comparison, can explain the knowledge I am using to inform my thinking and identify the sources of my supporting evidence and the justification for using it …
>
> … There seems to be an imbalance between their domains. Their ability to manage the interplay between intuitive and rational judgement and between theoretical and professional craft knowledge appears limited. Their weaknesses are often in relation to conscious decision-making (intentionality), knowing what matters (saliency) and timing, anticipating and pacing (temporality).

Maeve concluded that, despite her colleagues' well-developed relationship domain, they could not offer skilled companionship in an expert way. Maeve was right. The skilled companion needs all the domains to be able to offer evidence-based, person-centred care. For example, for mutuality (working with, in partnership) to be fully effective, all the other processes are prerequisite. Without *saliency* and *temporality*, how will practitioners know what are the most important, significant things to attend to, for example, developing trust in the relationship? And how will they know when the time is right to take a particular action that is likely to develop that trust?

Maeve wondered whether she had been able to develop skilled companionship better than her past colleagues just because she had been working longer in this field, but she concluded that perhaps her colleagues had not learned to integrate new practical or theoretical knowledge, over time, to 'form tacit knowledge and use it intuitively in their practice'.

> *M:* Another reason [could] be that they do not understand … how craft knowledge is actually created and how a practitioner's knowledge domains can be developed … They seem to think to increase one's knowledge you just take it from someone like me or read something and then one automatically has new knowledge … They do not appear to appreciate that to acquire new knowledge you need to process it fully. You have to integrate the theoretical knowledge with practical knowledge (know-how) to form tacit knowledge. When they encountered new things or a difficulty, their first instinct seemed to be to ask me to explain the new thing or solve their problem for them by telling them what to do.

This seeming inability to blend professional knowledges, through a process of systematic critique, might lead to less than optimal care, as tentatively suggested in Kate's account of her experience of hospital appointments and district nurses. There is more robust evidence in Binnie and Titchen's (1999) and Titchen's (2000) studies that nurses who were characterised as 'passing acquaintances' to their patients and families were not giving person-centred care. They were experienced as kind, but always busy with no time to really listen to and engage with them – very much as Kate experienced the district nurses. With skilful facilitation that came to be called critical companionship, they were helped to become skilled companions who were valued by patients and families.

They make me feel I have something to live for. It's the way they talk to me, the time they take to explain, being nice to me (Binnie & Titchen 1999, p. 186).

We really valued the honesty and patience with which you discussed the possibilities of medical intervention with us. You showed great skill in approaching these issues in a way that neither interfered with our choices nor left us feeling alone with the decisions we took. We felt happy with the eventual choice that allowed Harry a peaceful and dignified death (ibid., p. 180).

Critical companionship (Titchen 2001b) is a person-centred strategy for helping practitioners to understand the nature of their professional knowledge base, to create new professional craft knowledge from their practice and to blend and shape/influence their knowledges, as shown in Figure 7.1. We will return to this, but first we continue Maeve's story to find out how she developed the capacity she describes above to create and blend knowledge in her practice.

MAEVE'S KNOWLEDGE CREATION AND BLENDING

The following quote from Maeve's portfolio shows the contribution of propositional knowledge to the development of her professional craft knowledge. This contribution came in the form of new language and frameworks that enabled her to investigate her practice.

Relating Titchen's (2000) conceptual frameworks to my clinical practice and understanding the language she used when explaining them, initially, seemed like an impossibility.

However, Maeve found that reflection, through action learning (McGill & Beaty 1998), helped develop her understanding:

I could really see, as we reflected at the end of each action learning set, the various domains of knowledge and learning strategies that had been used and how they were actually used. This enabled me to get a real grasp and understanding of what I had been trying to read in terms of the conceptual frameworks and structured reflection (refer to Johns 2001; Titchen 2000).

... Now I feel the language used and my understanding of the conceptual frameworks ... is embedded in my knowledge and practice such that it is a vital and integral part of my professional craft knowledge ... Compiling and selecting material for inclusion in my portfolio, to demonstrate my expertise, brought me deep into my own subconscious and confronted me with the reality of how I and others perceive and understand my expertise ... Further I began to appreciate that to be able to articulate the value of nursing expertise one needed to be able to talk about it confidently and positively. To do that one needs the supporting evidence [and the language] ...

... What I have found through the experience of the project is that I can still be very critical of my own and others' clinical practice, but in a very constructive way. For example, using the conceptual frameworks of both skilled companionship and critical companionship I could see at an early stage in my journey that my reflective ability in terms of structured reflection and critique was not as good as it could be. I could equally see how I could address those issues. If someone challenged me now to explain my own expertise or even to analyse someone else's, as an expert I feel I could, not only articulate my thoughts clearly because I have frameworks and languages to help me to do so, but also I feel I could identify aspects of that expertise that may require development.

Since the completion of the project, we have further investigated, by e-mail and telephone, how Maeve blends self and professional. First, we examined her care of Joseph and his parents.

Angie (A): [Referring to Figure 7.1] How did you blend your knowledges to make your care person-centred?

M: While I brought all three forms of knowledge with me on my first visit to Joseph and his family, how I blended them together was shaped by the situation or context in which I found myself, particularly my understanding of what Joseph, Kate and Sean's specific needs were at that time, where they were at, balancing that against any risks and the need to prioritise actions to minimise any risk. I used my own personality to gain the information I needed in order to know the whole person I was trying to help, in this case that included Kate and Sean. I uncovered what kind of help they felt they needed. I blended my different forms of knowledge in such a way as to best help them. For example, when I initially visited, it was my propositional knowledge that played an important function, combined with my personal knowledge. This combination directed my decision to do the scan quickly to get an objective clinical diagnosis and help reduce anxiety levels. When I was doing the fuller assessment of Joseph, and initiating some treatment, I used more professional craft knowledge, combined with personal knowledge and, to a much lesser extent, propositional knowledge. Blending of the knowledges is, I feel, brought about by what you call 'professional artistry'. For me, this means looking at the whole person you're trying to help, asking what kind of help they need, where they are at, and then shaping the knowledges or weaving them together to help the patient and/or carer to get the best of it, to help them cope with where they are at, at that particular time.

A: How did you check out the validity of the knowledges and the blend and their usefulness in your work with Joseph and his family?

M: By critically reflecting when in the actual situations and after my visits to Joseph's home, particularly when writing up his notes. I also checked these things by discussing my thoughts and actions with other nurses and other professionals involved in Joseph's care. In particular, I shared the knowledges I was using with the hospice nurse who had been involved with Joseph and his family for a number of years. She was very much in agreement with my understanding of the case and the approach I was taking. When I spoke to the urologist this was another opportunity in which I was able to validate the knowledges I was using, their blend and usefulness. He agreed not only with my clinical diagnosis, but also with the actions I had initiated. The propositional knowledge and professional craft knowledge I had used were further validated through the results of the clinical tests carried out by the urologist.

A: How do you know that the knowledge/blend had the impact you intended, in terms of being person-centred?

M: First, Kate and Sean's level of anxiety was visibly reduced. Second, Joseph's residual urine volumes decreased and he gradually began to improve. Third, Kate and Sean actively began to seek information/advice from me and when upset or even angry about something they would phone me and share it with me and trust me to act on their behalf. Fourth, Joseph began to actually attempt to speak to me and even touch me when I visited him.

Our search 'within' is enough for the moment. Unlike the search for the bull 'out there', our search 'within' has been meaningful. Our tree of knowledges is beginning to bear fruit! Effortlessly!

Now, it is time to turn these insights into theoretical principles. We can do this by putting together the analytical frameworks (Figs 7.1 and 7.2) that we have already examined, and creating Figure 7.3.

This figure is a dynamic, transformative model. Imagine that the three types of knowledge are twirling simultaneously, rather like cake-mixer attachments. Imagine, too, that the skilled companionship model in the centre of the blend is also whirling. The result is that the professional blends all types of knowledge and creates different, unique blends or patterns for the particular patient, situation, context. It is always different. Taking the cake-making imagery further, imagine a particular aspect of theoretical (propositional knowledge) as brandy which is poured into the mixer (cf. MacLeod 1990). Blended by the professional artistry of the skilled companion, the brandy is physically transformed; never again can it be separate and poured back into the bottle, but its distinctive flavour permeates the cake and is clearly recognisable. This can be thought of as a kind of alchemy or transformation of theoretical knowledge into practice knowledge. Another image that might help to understand this seemingly mysterious blending is looking at Figure 7.3 as a kaleidoscope. With each patient, the professional turns it to transform the pattern of the crystals; they are the same crystals, but their form and balance have been rearranged. So it seems to be with the practitioner, drawing on different aspects of the different knowledges and creating something new each time. It is not just one pattern or one blend that the person-centred practitioner offers, but an endless number of variations and diversity. But there is always one constancy at the point of balance, the place of stillness, at the centre of the model: the patient/client–practitioner relationship.

So we return to professional artistry. We suggest that it is professional artistry that enables the creation of the right blend, pattern or balance for each unique interaction and intervention. It is difficult to put into words. We mentioned it earlier as the balance and interplay between the skilled companionship domains and between rational thinking and intuition, within the

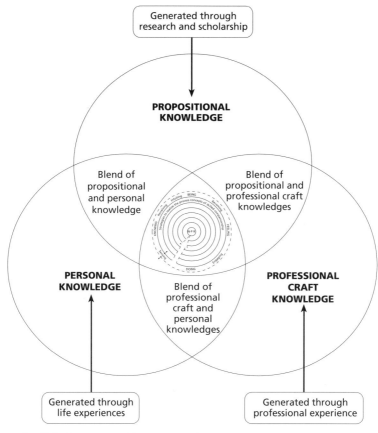

Figure 7.3   Skilled companionship: a strategy for blending self and professional knowledges through professional artistry

therapeutic use of self. Titchen and Higgs (2001) took that work further in their description of professional artistry as taking the forms of synchronicity, balance, attunement and interplay; as if it were a jazz improvisation, where professional artistry emerges through a conversation with different aspects or players of the professional self. They proposed that professional artistry is a blend of:

- practitioner qualities, such as connoisseurship, bodily, emotional and spiritual intelligences, passion, adventurousness, courage, awareness of self, others and context
- practice skills, e.g. expert critical appreciation, ability to disclose or express what has been observed, perceived or done
- *metacognitive* awareness (i.e. thinking about thinking, reasoning about reasoning)

- creative imagination processes, e.g. imagining how we can transform ourselves, others, organisations, professions or the outcomes of personalised, unique patient/client interventions and creative strategies to achieve them.

By using cognitive, intuitive and sense modes of perception, professional artistry enables the practitioner to:

- mediate propositional, professional craft and personal knowledges, bodily, emotional and spiritual intelligences in the use of applied and clinical sciences, through professional judgement
- realise practical principles
- use whole self therapeutically, facilitatively and creatively.

Professional artistry can be facilitated through critical companionship, a strategy that we mentioned earlier, as a means for helping practitioners to become skilled companions. Now we look in more detail at how critical companionship works.

FACILITATING UNDERSTANDING OF THE NATURE AND GENERATION OF KNOWLEDGES AND THEIR BLENDING

We have developed an extended skilled companionship framework which shows how self and professional knowledges can be blended through professional artistry. Understanding and being able to practise this artistry can lead to approaches to health and social care that are evidence-based and person-centred. We propose that, if practitioners understand the ontology and epistemology of person-centred practice, as shown in Figure 7.3, then they can better develop a deeper knowing of their core values, of their human qualities and attributes and of their role interactions with others, and blend this knowing with their propositional and professional craft knowledge to deliver evidence-based, person-centred care. Based on this premise, which is justified through Maeve's story and elsewhere (RCN 2002), we show how critical companionship can support practitioners' investigating their own practices, and how practitioners can prepare themselves for becoming critical companions to colleagues. But first we need to look at the derivation of prerequisite knowledges, to understand how practitioners use different knowledges to create new knowledge from and in their practice (Titchen & Ersser 2001).

These prerequisite knowledges are:

- experiential personal knowledge, such as aesthetic, intuitive and embodied knowledge or ontological knowing, derived through the senses
- ontological knowing derived through socialisation, such as our core values, ethical/moral knowledge, knowledge of our personal qualities

and attributes, and of ourselves in interaction with others within a variety of roles
• propositional knowledge derived through research and scholarship.

Critical companions, in relation to a specific situation, raise to consciousness (and draw out) the above knowledges, relevant to the case, for critical review. Just as Angie posed questions to Maeve, so companions ask questions to help practitioners consider how they acquire, use and create their holistic practice knowledge and how they check its validity, its blend and usefulness in practice. Companions then help practitioners to see how these knowledges can be used to create new professional craft knowledge about how to deliver evidence-based, person-centred care. This knowledge creation can be done in at least two ways:

• research/theory is actively tested in practice for verifiability and usefulness by practitioners (deductive knowledge creation)
• informed by the three forms of knowledge, practitioners observe and make sense of their person-centred practices over time (inductive knowledge creation).

The first knowledge creation process is the one most easily articulated by practitioners.

> *M:* My professional craft knowledge is created within myself as a result of applying and testing, in clinical practice, the theories and research evidence that I have formally gained. When I read a theory in a book I feel the need to test it out in reality. It has been my experience, even when I studied art, that when I did test out what I had read the result was always different from that in the book. For example, in my art book it would state that if you mix yellow and blue you get green. When I did so the green colour I got was always a very different shade compared to the colour displayed in the book. When I came into nursing I brought with me that sense of having to test out things for myself. Everything I learned I wanted to apply and test it with the individual, the patient. My experience has been that in doing so, I always have to reshape the theory to suit the patient's unique needs. In doing so, with each patient, I learn something new which contributes continuously to what is now my professional craft knowledge.

The critical companion facilitates all the above processes by helping the practitioner to develop the cognitive, metacognitive and artistry processes necessary for such work. Critical companions understand these processes and are able, using a range of practical strategies, to help others develop their knowledge use, acquisition and creation in a conscious, critical way.

Critical companionship parallels skilled companionship in that it has the same relationship, rationality–intuitive and use-of-self domains. These domains are put into practice using the same or similar strategies which are shaped by the new contexts and roles of the people in the relationship. It is through a person-centred approach to facilitating the other's learning that the critical companion models the facilitative use of self, not only giving the other a direct experience of skilled companionship, but also articulating the processes and strategies that he or she is using. Around skilled companionship at the heart of the critical companionship framework is added the facilitation domain and strategies which transform the enabling relationship into a critical one.

Maeve's working with Brendan not only provided her with exemplary critical companionship, it also alerted her to the need to become a critical companion herself. Through the experience of using the skilled companionship framework to analyse her own and then her colleagues' practice, Maeve discovered that she needed to transfer the person-centred skills with patients to working with her colleagues, just as Titchen (2000) found. Before the project, Maeve had determined what her colleagues needed in order to develop their knowledge. She had then 'spoon-fed' them information and given them research articles to read. During the project, Maeve realised that, just as she needed to know where her patients are, so that she could accompany them on their illness journeys, so she had to do the same with her colleagues on their learning journeys. She came to see that she could be more effective if she used the critical companionship processes that Brendan was modelling for her.

> Using Titchen's (2001b) critical companionship framework in the form of a matrix (RCN 1999), I found, through an analysis of myself as a critical companion, that while my relationship and rationality–intuitive domains were good, I was not strong in terms of my facilitation concepts. I was effective in consciousness-raising and problematisation, but I needed to strengthen my reflection and critique concepts … I also need to strengthen my use of certain facilitation strategies, particularly more forms for articulating my craft knowledge and to use critical dialogue more confidently.

Although, for the purposes of the project, Brendan helped Maeve gather evidence of her expertise, he was also modelling how to do this in a rigorous way in everyday practice, and how to subject evidence from multiple sources to systematic critique, critical control and review. The overall results were that, first, Maeve felt affirmed in giving genuinely evidence-based and person-centred care, and second, she enhanced her blend of self and professional in her developing role of critical companion to her colleagues.

CONCLUSION

In this chapter we have offered a possible answer to the question, 'How can understanding the nature and generation of knowledge facilitate a person-centred approach to health and social care?' We constructed a possible answer by attending to the wisdom illustrated in the poem which led us to a search for the subjective within Maeve's person-centred practice. We have transformed the subjective, using analytic tools developed through research and scholarship, into a contextualised, potentially transferable form. This form is a dynamic, extended, skilled companionship framework, as a strategy for blending self and professional knowledges, through professional artistry. We have described how mature, self-aware, sensitive and skilled practitioners can deliver evidence-based, yet unique, personalised patient care that the patient wants and needs. They do this by blending self and professional through an inextricable twining of propositional, professional craft and personal knowledges. This may be accomplished through professional artistry, as described here. We conclude that the development of such artistry can be facilitated through critical companionship strategies within any experiential learning context (e.g. clinical supervision and action learning).

Critical companionship relates to skilled companionship through parallel relationships, knowledges, knowledge creation processes and professional artistry, hence the Russian doll analogy alluded to earlier. The term 'companion' was chosen with care, to denote a relationship that is like a friendship, but is not (Titchen 2000). Unlike friendship, there is a mutual expectation of parting at the end of the professional encounter. Most friendships do not work like that; neither are they set up formally for offering professional help for a particular health-care-related purpose.

Through the relationship with the practitioner, the companion models the ontology and epistemology of professional practice, articulates the cognitive, metacognitive and artistry involved and nurtures their development in the other. Through the extra facilitation domain, the critical companion enables the skilled companion to become a researcher and a transformer of his or her practice and context, raising to consciousness the blending of self and professional and the entwinement of knowledges acquired, used and created through the giving of person-centred care. And so 'the dead trees become alive'.

ACKNOWLEDGEMENTS

The verses of the poem were obtained from http://www.cs.sfu.ca/people/ResearchStaff/jamie/personal/10_Bulls/1.html.

The assistance of Professor Brendan McCormack of the University of Ulster and Director of Nursing Research at the Royal Hospitals, Belfast, in the preparation of this chapter is much appreciated.

REFERENCES

Benner, P. (1984). *From Novice to Expert: Excellence and Power in Clinical Nursing Practice.* London: Addison-Wesley.

Binnie, A. & Titchen, A. (1999). *Freedom to Practise: The Development of Patient-Centred Nursing* (J. Lathlean, ed.). Oxford: Butterworth-Heinemann.

Bottorff, J. (1991). The lived experience of being comforted by a nurse. *Phenomenology and Pedagogy*, **9**, 237–52.

Boykin, A. & Schoenhofer, S. (1993). *Nursing as Caring: A Model for Transforming Practice.* New York: National League for Nursing Press.

Brown, L. (1986). The experience of care: patient perspectives. *Topics in Clinical Nursing*, **8**(2), 56–62.

Edwards, C. (2002). *Transformation of Opinion Within the Patient's Process of Reflection on Healthcare*. PhD thesis. University of Manchester: RCN Institute.

Eraut, M. (1994). *Developing Professional Knowledge and Competence*. London: Falmer Press.

Ersser, S. J. (1997). *Nursing as a Therapeutic Activity: An Ethnography*. Developments in Nursing and Health Care 14. Aldershot: Avebury.

Forrest, D. (1989). The experience of caring. *Journal of Advanced Nursing*, **14**, 815–23.

Freshwater, D. (1998). The philosopher's stone. In *Transforming Nursing Through Reflective Practice* (C. Johns & D. Freshwater, eds) pp. 177–84. Oxford: Blackwell Science.

Higgs, J. & Titchen, A. (2000). Knowledge and reasoning. In *Clinical Reasoning in the Health Professions*, 2nd edn (J. Higgs & M. Jones, eds) pp. 23–32. Oxford: Butterworth-Heinemann.

Higgs, J. & Titchen, A. (eds) (2001). *Professional Practice in Health, Education and the Creative Arts*. Oxford: Blackwell Science.

Johns, C. (2001). Reflective practice: revealing the art of caring. *International Journal of Nurse Practice*, **7**, 237–45.

MacLeod, M. (1990). *Experience in Everyday Nursing Practice: A Study of 'Experienced' Ward Sisters*. Doctoral thesis. Edinburgh: University of Edinburgh.

Manley, K. & McCormack, B. (1997). *Exploring Expert Practice*. MSc nursing distance learning module. London: Royal College of Nursing.

McGill, I. & Beaty, L. (1998). *Action Learning: A Guide for Professional, Management and Educational Development*. London: Kogan Page.

McMahon, R. & Pearson, A. (1991). *Nursing as Therapy*. London: Chapman & Hall.

Parse, R. R., Coyne, A. B. & Smith, M. J. (1985). *Nursing Research: Qualitative Methods*. Bowie, MD: Brady Communications.

RCN (1999). *Realising Clinical Effectiveness and Clinical Governance Through Clinical Supervision*. Royal College of Nursing Institute open learning pack (critical companionship matrix in Module 1, p. 85). Abingdon: Radcliffe Medical Press.

RCN (2002). *Expertise in Practice Project: Final Report*. Practice Development Function. London: Royal College of Nursing.

Reps, P. (comp.) (1957). *Zen Flesh, Zen Bones*. Boston: Charles E. Tuttle.

Taylor, B. J. (1992). Relieving pain through ordinariness in nursing: a phenomenologic account of a comforting nurse–patient encounter. *Advances in Nursing Science*, **15**(1), 33–43.

Titchen, A. (2000). *Professional Craft Knowledge in Patient-Centred Nursing and the Facilitation of its Development*. University of Oxford DPhil thesis. Oxford: Ashdale Press.

Titchen, A. (2001a). Skilled companionship in professional practice. In *Practice Knowledge and Expertise in the Health Professions* (J. Higgs & A. Titchen, eds) pp. 69–79. Oxford: Butterworth-Heinemann.

Titchen, A. (2001b). Critical companionship: a conceptual framework for developing expertise. In *Practice Knowledge and Expertise in the Health Professions* (J. Higgs & A. Titchen, eds) pp. 80–90. Oxford: Butterworth-Heinemann.

Titchen, A. & Ersser, S. (2001). Explicating, creating and validating professional craft knowledge. In *Practice Knowledge and Expertise in the Health Professions* (J. Higgs & A. Titchen, eds) pp. 48–56. Oxford: Butterworth-Heinemann.

Titchen, A. & Higgs, J. (2001). Towards professional artistry and creativity in practice. In *Professional Practice in Health, Education and the Creative Arts* (J. Higgs & A. Titchen, eds) pp. 273–90. Oxford: Blackwell Science.

8

The use and generation of practice knowledge in the context of regulating systems and moral frameworks

Julius Sim and Barbara Richardson

INTRODUCTION

In this chapter we seek to explore the way in which practice in health care, and the knowledge that underpins it, can be subject to forces and processes that potentially constrain professional activity. We argue that the 'ideal' of clinical decision-making, with its emphasis on rationality, is influenced by a variety of sometimes conflicting sources of knowledge and modes of thinking. We consider the role of various regulatory frameworks, such as resource allocation policies, research governance requirements and codes of ethics, in shaping and constraining practice. Finally, the relationship of professional knowledge and practice to moral and other values is analysed, and recommendations for professional practice and education are made.

THE IDEAL OF CLINICAL DECISION-MAKING

Professional practice may be seen as a rational process of clinical reasoning, leading to a treatment or management decision that is synthesised from an analysis of theory and clinical information (Fig. 8.1). *Theoretical knowledge* may originate from general theory in academic disciplines such as psychology, sociology or physiology. Alternatively, it may be derived from the specific extant knowledge of professions, such as the models of care developed in

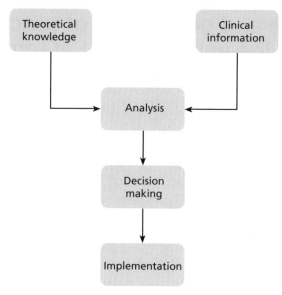

Figure 8.1 A model of clinical decision-making

the disciplines of nursing (McKenna 1997) or occupational therapy (Hagedorn 1999). In either case, theory may be based purely on theoretical reasoning or may, in addition, be grounded in empirical research; in the latter case, knowledge might be described as evidence-based. It will also be, in part, formulated from the past experience of the individual. *Clinical information* is derived from the specific clinical situation. It may be based on features relating directly to the individual client, such as signs and symptoms, or it may take the form of contextual information, such as the social and cultural background of the client.

By a process of analysis, theoretical knowledge is applied to this clinical information (i.e. the information is analysed in terms of theory), and a decision is reached about professional action. Following consideration of the circumstances and inherent constraints of the particular situation (resources available, patient or practitioner preferences, etc.), the decision may be further amended before it is implemented.

The process may work in a more complex way than just suggested. There may, for example, be an interplay between information and analysis. As the result of an initial analysis, additional information may be sought, leading to further analysis, or there may be feedback between decision-making and implementation, as various clinical hypotheses are tested (Jones et al 2000). Additionally, the practitioner may be conscious of the process of decision-making and the way in which knowledge is being used, and may adapt or regulate the way in which it occurs, through a process of metacognition (Higgs & Jones 2000). That is, the practitioner may analyse not only the

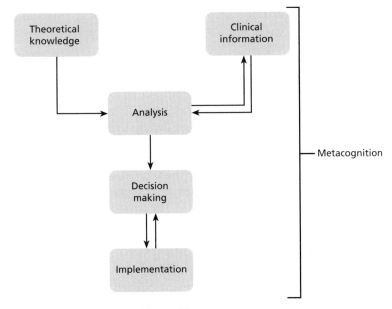

Figure 8.2   Metacognition in decision-making

conclusion arrived at but also the way in which it was reached, and such reflection may cause a reappraisal of the way in which this or future decisions are made. This is particularly likely to occur in situations that permit unhurried, strategic decision-making, rather than circumstances in which an immediate decision is required. These processes are illustrated in Figure 8.2.

In essence, it may be debated whether one's theoretical knowledge drives the attention given to information presented in the clinical situation, or whether experience of clinical situations drives the development of a framework of theoretical knowledge, or whether the two processes occur in parallel; however, this model remains one of a rational, linear process of logical reasoning, grounded in putatively objective facts drawn from the clinical situation.

Limitations

This ideal model of clinical decision-making has, however, a number of shortcomings. First, it does not necessarily represent the reality of everyday clinical practice. Decision-making may occur through other processes, such as clinical intuition or the use of standardised routines that may exist in a particular clinical setting. In the process, practitioners may draw upon other sources of knowledge than formally acknowledged theory. Private as well as public sources of knowledge may be utilised. Decision-making in everyday practice may thus differ somewhat from the process depicted in an ideal theoretical model. Accordingly, in parallel with findings in the sociology of science (Woolgar 1988), the ideal model may represent the reconstructed rather than the actual logic of practice.

Second, the gathering and utilisation of factual information, and the status of such information, are more problematic than is acknowledged. Facts are socially constructed, according to an individual's values and presuppositions about the nature of the external world; they are created, not discovered. What counts as a fact, or which facts are deemed relevant, or the priority that is attached to particular facts, is subject to a number of subjective influences. Hence, the way that factual information contributes to clinical decision-making is conditioned by the nature of the theoretical knowledge brought to bear and, most crucially, by the values and experiences of the individual decision-maker.

Third, clinical decision-making is subject to a number of flaws of reasoning, often referred to as heuristic biases (Sprent 1988). These may cause certain aspects of a situation to be unduly salient in the practitioner's mind, or to assume a disproportionate importance in the process of reaching a decision (Sim 1995). A robust and more practical model of decision-making must make room for this slippage from the ideal, acknowledging the fact that practical decision-making is intimately related to and conditioned by the situation in which it occurs.

Finally, although social context and social processes may form part of the data upon which clinical reasoning is based, there is no acknowledgement in the model that the process of clinical decision-making is itself subject to these and other forces. A final decision is intrinsically tied to the particular context in which it occurs.

Sources of knowledge

Within professional practice, there are a number of sources of knowledge upon which practitioners can draw. The tenets of evidence-based practice (EBP) place greatest emphasis on knowledge derived from empirical research, or more specifically, empirical research that can be shown to be methodologically sound and capable of being generalised to normal patterns of practice. As yet, however, there is little evidence of this being fully applied in practice (Closs & Lewin 1998). In addition, practitioners make use of experiential knowledge, accumulated from their own everyday practice, or various forms of traditional knowledge, gained from colleagues (Higgs & Titchen 1995). These empirical or experiential sources of knowledge depend upon an individual's manner of observing and responding to events in the outside world. Another source of knowledge, rationalism, comes from within the individual and depends upon theoretical reasoning rather than on data from the real world. Here, conclusions are reached a priori (according to the conceptual and logical relationships believed to exist between certain propositions), rather than a posteriori (according to observed facts in the external world). This type of a priori understanding is important in developing models or theories of practice, or identifying hypotheses that can subsequently be put to an empirical test, as these models or hypotheses may represent a departure from or an alternative to the usual way of viewing the world. A similar type of reasoning underlies ethical decision-making, which relies ultimately on judgements about how the world should be, rather than observations about how the world actually is.

An example or two may clarify these ideas. A health care profession may conceive of its work in terms of a particular model of care, based, perhaps, on notions of client independence. However, reflection on the nature and definition of illness or disability may suggest that there is a logical relationship between illness and the notion of personhood. Accordingly, an alternative model of care might be proposed that has its roots in a fundamentally different conceptualisation of illness, and this model would have derived not so much from the external facts of illness (i.e. observing people who are ill) but from theoretical reflection upon the conceptual basis of illness as an abstract, unobservable entity. Similarly, a practitioner faced with a particular ethical conflict will seek resources to assist in its resolution. A satisfactory resolution cannot, however, come from studying actions that have been taken in the past in such situations, or from surveying the views of colleagues. Empirical facts may well be important in terms of framing an ethical question (e.g. in identifying that a confidence has been broken, or that a form of harm is likely to occur), but they cannot on their own deliver an ethical conclusion. This follows the principle 'ought cannot be derived from is', laid down by the 18th-century philosopher David Hume (Harrison 1976). Rather than seek to deduce a moral conclusion from the facts of the case, the practitioner must relate these facts to general ethical concepts and principles (such as outlined in the following section) and consider their logical relationship (e.g. whether a particular action would be compatible with one ethical principle or in contravention of another) in the process of decision-making. Moreover, judgements as to the relative importance of certain ethical principles are likely to be required (whether one such principle should be given precedence over another) and here again the *actual* state of the world is not the issue.

The status of these various forms of knowledge will vary in different contexts. According to Turner and Whitfield (1999), clinicians accord a higher value to received knowledge, as represented by their undergraduate teaching, than to papers in scientific journals. In contrast, advocates of EBP place the emphasis on research-based knowledge (Charles 2002). Hence, in the popular hierarchy of evidence for clinical effectiveness, evidence from randomised controlled trials and systematic reviews lies at or near the top (Bury 1998). A popular definition of EBP portrays it as 'the conscientious, explicit and judicious use of current best evidence in making decisions about the care of individual patients' (Sackett et al 1996, p. 71). Sources of knowledge are not necessarily irreconcilable, however. Hence, Sackett et al further state that the 'practice of evidence based medicine means integrating individual clinical expertise with the best available external clinical evidence from systematic research' (ibid., p. 71). Thus, when taking action as part of either clinical or ethical decision-making, the practitioner may enlist a variety of forms of knowledge, some of which may be grounded in empirical evidence, and others of which may derive from more intuitive sources. (Chapter 9 presents further discussion of EBP and associated issues.)

SPHERES OF ACCOUNTABILITY OF THE PRACTITIONER

In the discharge of their professional work, practitioners are subject to a number of demands. In the first instance, there are what might be termed *internal* demands. These are requirements to which professionals consider themselves to be subject in terms of their perceived professional responsibility. Thus, there is a requirement to treat or manage the individual client effectively, to the best of one's professional skill – what might be termed *demands of professional competence*. Similarly, from the perspective of morality (or ethics), there is a requirement to respect the individual client's autonomy and welfare, and to balance the needs of different clients in a way that is just and non-discriminatory – what might be termed *demands of ethics*. Table 8.1 shows some fundamental ethical principles that generate moral requirements for individuals in the practice of health care. These principles command a high degree of universality. Although they may be expressed in different terms, the relative priority accorded to them may change over time, and the specific conclusions derived from them may vary, these principles tend to underlie most secular and religious systems of morality, both past and present (Gillon 1994).

Various professional groups may appear to claim a particular ethics, as suggested by certain uses of the terms 'medical ethics', 'nursing ethics', and

Table 8.1 Basic ethical principles

Principle	Description
Beneficence	The positive requirement to promote the interests and well-being of others and protect them from harm
Non-maleficence	The negative requirement not to cause harm to others
Respect for autonomy	The requirement to protect and/or to promote the self-determination of others
Respect for persons	The requirement to respect the dignity and individuality of others, and not to treat them merely as means to an end
Justice	The requirement to treat others fairly, such that differential treatment of others must be morally justifiable in relation to morally relevant differences between them

(From Sim (1997), with permission of Butterworth-Heinemann.)

the like, and by the fact that each profession has a particular ethical code. This might imply that there is a type of moral knowledge that is specific to a certain professional group, and that consequently those outside the discipline concerned are to some degree unequipped to evaluate or even interpret moral judgements made within the discipline. However, although certain ways of ethical thinking may be *characteristic* of a profession, in that its members may generally agree on certain basic moral values and may apply them to concrete cases in a similar way, that is not to say that such ways of thinking are in any sense the *prerogative* of that profession. Ethical principles and methods of ethical decision-making are open to all, and membership of a particular professional discipline cannot in itself provide unique moral insights or confer a form of moral authority. Of course, being in a particular profession may place one in situations in which experience (and thus perhaps expertise) in ethical decision-making is developed. However, in such a situation membership of the profession is a means to, not a precondition of, such experience.

Meanwhile, there are also *external* demands placed on the practitioner. There are *legal demands*: the civil and criminal law place certain prescriptions and proscriptions on the professional, concerning such issues as negligence, confidentiality and contractual obligations related to employment. These demands relate predominantly to the context of the individual patient or client. Additionally, there are what one can call *institutional demands*. These are frameworks of requirements emanating from institutional or statutory bodies, which direct practice in the context of more general patterns of practice implementation, relating mainly to questions of clinical effectiveness and resource allocation. Thus, in the USA practitioners are required to work according to the stipulations of third-party payers such as Medicaid or Medicare, which permit reimbursement in relation to specified diagnostic-related groups. A consequence of this is that clinical expertise, and therefore knowledge, may have opportunity to develop in those diagnostic groups that have become the preferred choices for resource allocation. In the UK, the National Health Service (NHS) has established clinical governance frameworks within which clinicians must work, and the National Institute for Clinical Effectiveness has the power to determine which treatments can be given within the NHS for certain diagnoses. Again, these requirements placed on contemporary clinical practice may constrain practitioners in their work and prevail against development of knowledge outside these confines, which may be needed to respond to changing health care needs. Another source of institutional demands is the profession as a collectivity, which creates obligations with respect to professional codes of conduct and the need to maintain or promote professional autonomy, the interpretation of which may be out of step with contemporary health needs. An example is the apparent challenge to professional autonomy presented by working in teams.

The examples of institutional demands given hitherto concern the application of professional knowledge. However, it can be seen that such demands may also influence the generation of professional knowledge. In addition, funding bodies, through their control of the purse strings and stipulation of specific protocols, can present regulatory frameworks that largely determine which research questions can be investigated. Institutional Review Boards in the USA, or Research Ethics Committees in the UK, can strongly influence which types of research are sanctioned to proceed, based on considerations of favoured or disfavoured methodologies, with little challenge or concern for any moral argument underpinning them.

With regard to individual practice, these sets of demands can overlap. For example, demands of clinical effectiveness may overlap with those of ethics, in that there is a moral obligation to practise to the best of one's ability (that is, using one's utmost knowledge and skill). Similarly, institutional demands imposed through a code of practice or resource allocation guidelines will generally be claimed to have a basis in moral notions such as beneficence or justice. In contrast, there may be conflicts between different sets of demands, and these are particularly likely to become apparent when individual and collective interests are in tension. Resource allocation policies or clinical governance requirements are framed with categories of clients in mind, whereas the practitioner may be confronted with a specific client whose clinical needs, or whose likelihood of therapeutic benefit, are not those of the 'average' client.

SPECIFIC AREAS OF CONFLICT
Resource allocation

Issues of resource allocation have always exerted a strong influence on the nature and pattern of professional practice, although practitioners themselves have not always acknowledged this. Broadly, resource allocation has to do with the distribution of health care resources, in terms of what health care interventions should be available, to whom, and in what quantity. Decisions made in this context will sooner or later involve a judgement as to which of two clients should receive a particular service, or at least who should receive it first. Resource allocation is therefore often conceptualised in terms of the health care cake: a slice for one person may mean no slice for another, or a larger slice for one implies a smaller slice for another. Underlying this analogy is the long-established view that health care resources are finite but health needs are infinite: 'the appetite for medical care *vient en mangeant*' (Powell 1976, p. 27). An additional underlying assumption concerns how the cake is conceptualised, whether it is considered to be aimed predominantly to provide primary, secondary or tertiary health care services, raising questions of how priority decisions are made.

Resource allocation in health care can occur on two levels. Macroallocation relates to decisions taken in respect of different types of goods or services (either within the health sphere or between this and other spheres) and in respect of certain *categories* of patient. In contrast, microallocation relates to decisions taken in respect of the patient, or of small groups of patients, and usually concerns individual *cases* (Sim 1997).

Policies relating to macroallocation may be formulated by statutory bodies (e.g. the National Institute for Clinical Excellence in the UK) or by institutions such as insurance companies and other third-party payers (e.g. Medicaid in the USA). Policies of microallocation are likely to arise at the level of a particular institution, unit or individual practitioner. Although not always fully aware of it, individual professionals working in public health care are almost certain to be practising within a context of macroallocation. Equally, and again without their necessarily being aware of it, they are likely to operate microallocation policies, in terms of such everyday decisions as how long to treat individual patients, where to place patients on a waiting list, whether to take a hands-on approach or one based on education and advice, and such like.

Three key issues underlying resource allocation are *effectiveness* (the degree to which an intervention produces benefits), *efficiency* (the relationship between the benefits of an intervention and the cost of its provision) and *equity* (the fairness with which resources are allocated between individual clients). The last of these concerns the principle of justice, outlined in Table 8.1. Justice does not require that each person should receive the same quantity of a resource or benefits: equity does not assume equality. However, it does require that individuals should be treated differently only on the basis of morally relevant considerations. If differential treatment is based on morally irrelevant criteria, such as race, religion or personal preference, it constitutes discrimination. Some criteria, such as age, can be morally relevant in one situation and morally irrelevant in another.

The most obvious criterion for resource allocation is that of need. It is generally accepted that those in most need have the strongest claim on resources, such that need is considered a morally relevant factor in allocating care. However, this provision requires the needs of individual clients to be assessed in not only absolute but also relative terms. Because not all needs are amenable to intervention at the level of health care, it is common practice to focus not on the individual's health-related needs per se, but on his or her capacity to benefit from health care intervention. This creates a subset – needs that are capable of being met within a health care system.

Recognising both the necessity and the difficulty of such needs assessment, health economists have developed devices such as the quality-adjusted life-year (QALY). The QALY seeks to measure a health-related benefit in units that represent both the quantity and the quality of that benefit. Thus, a year of healthy life expectancy would be rated at 1 QALY, and a year of relatively unhealthy life expectancy would be rated at some figure less than 1 (Williams 1985). The underlying rationale for the QALY is that 'it is no longer relevant to measure life expectancy in unadjusted years because a single year of perfect health, in terms of utility, may be equivalent to more than one year of impaired health' (Edgar et al 1998, p. 37).

The precise ratings of various states of health are generated by periodically surveying members of the public, asking them what hypothetical trade-offs they would be prepared to make between the quality of life and its quantity in certain specified situations. For a particular intervention, its QALY value is the difference in the number of QALYs accrued with the intervention and the number accrued either without the intervention or with an alternative intervention (Sim 1997). QALYs are calculated very much with the 'typical' patient in mind, and to that extent may be of limited use in making treatment choices about individuals. Indeed, it would be morally remiss not to take due account of the particular characteristics and circumstances of each patient when making such decisions. However, providing that due account is taken of their generality, QALYs may be regarded as a useful part of clinical decision-making by managing authorities and, as Dougherty (1994) points out, QALYs may provide patients with a consistent, systematic means of choosing between the benefits of different treatments, and may thereby assist autonomous choice.

Although framed with the intention of maximising health care benefits, resource allocation policies can create problems for health professionals in their everyday practice. At the level of macroallocation, policies are premised on the notion of aggregate benefit: to maximise the benefits for patients in general. These policies do not always allow for atypical patients who go against the overall trend. Thus, in a discussion of problems that may arise from the use of diagnosis-related groups (DRGs) and the provisions of the 1982 Health Care Financing Administration ruling in the USA that specifies 3 hours of therapy a day, Neuhaus (1988, p. 291) comments:

It is difficult to set realistic priorities that have some meaning for the patient when the patient's length of hospital stay has been determined on the basis of a diagnostic category that denies the individuality of patients in general as well as the specific needs of that particular person.

The individual practitioner must seek to reconcile the needs of individual clients with the requirement to work within a broader context of effective and efficient health care delivery. However, resource allocation policies, which may work against the interests of some individual clients, are often reinforced by a number of bureaucratic and institutional mechanisms, creating considerable pressure on the practitioner to conform with established practices.

Much the same conflict may arise at a more local level, where the need to deliver effective care across a caseload may be at odds with the need to serve an individual client's needs. What is most efficient to the service as a whole may not be what is most effective for the individual client. Clinical and managerial perspectives may be brought into conflict. This conflict is made all the harder to resolve because, on the one hand, each perspective is morally valid, in that there is a need to serve the interests of both the individual and the collectivity, but on the other hand clinicians and managers characteristically feel that their primary moral responsibility is to the individual patient and patients as a group, respectively.

A potentially more troubling conflict occurs where the perceived needs of the client are in tension with certain vested interests of an institution or a statutory body. A health care provider might wish to place restrictions on the care that can be given, for reasons that concern solely the financial or other interests of that organisation. For example, certain treatment costs may not be reimbursable to the provider, or the care of certain patients may not be sufficiently profitable, or may not accord with some sense of corporate profile. The individual practitioner working in such a context may feel that his or her practice is restricted for reasons that are not morally legitimate. In all of these examples it can be seen that the use, and thus the development, of professional knowledge can be potentially influenced or constrained.

Clinical governance and managed-care policies

In many countries resource allocation is seen to be central to clinical governance and becomes manifest in polces of managed-care pathways, which aim to optimise the use of health care services and health care space (Weiner et al 2002). Pathways of care based upon norms of recovery from specific disease presentations would appear to be a laudable way to ensure effective and equitable care and maximal progression rate through the system. However, discharge dates determined within such a system may be at odds with desirable levels of rehabilitation, unless the system's operational criteria take into account a range of levels and circumstances of functional outcome for individual clients. Lane (2000), for example, drew attention to the practical reality of the views cited above by Neuhaus (1988), when she described the issues of conflict that confront occupational therapists regarding the increased focus on client responsibility and choice and the decreasing time for rehabilitation prior to discharge. Such frameworks of practice, established through principles of clinical governance, can clearly constrain the way in which final rehabilitation needs are conceptualised. They may also influence perceptions of traditional professional profiles when, for example, occupational therapists are increasingly expected to take a lead in the coordination of discharge. In such situations, professional practice can be limited and the opportunity for the practice of professional knowledge can be undermined.

Professional codes

Professions operate, by definition, under the aegis of a code of ethics (Purtilo 1987). This is a set of requirements and/or guidelines as to the type of professional behaviour to be expected from members of the profession concerned. The internal demands of professional competence and of ethics to which the practitioner responds, as outlined earlier, are reflected in a more public and external form in a code of ethics. A code of ethics is intended to represent the consensus view of the profession, and admission to the profession at the conclusion of a qualifying course of training is usually conditional upon explicit or implicit acceptance of such a code. Equally, contravention of the requirements of the code may be the basis for removal from the profession.

For a code of ethics to be correctly described as such, it should relate to issues of a genuinely ethical nature (i.e. those concerning morality). Indeed, most codes do refer predominantly to questions of client welfare, which are of clear moral concern. However, codes of ethics may embody other considerations. These may, for example, relate to matters of professional etiquette or of professional self-interest, such as a concern for the public reputation of the profession. In fact, codes may be more specific in provisions relating to the profession's own interests than those relating to client welfare (Kultgen 1982). The interests of the professions do not necessarily match those of the public, even if one does not go so far as George Bernard Shaw, who argued that all professions are a conspiracy against the laity (Shaw 1946). Alternatively, some tenets of a code of ethics may concern legal considerations, which are not necessarily related to ethics in the strict sense of morality. Legal requirements do not automatically carry moral weight (Lyons 1984). A code of ethics therefore contains not only moral but also legal and professional requirements, which may or may not be grounded in ethics in the strict sense. For these reasons, it may in some cases be more appropriate to use the term 'code of professional conduct' when referring to these codes, rather than 'code of ethics'; the former term embraces this wider range of requirements, beyond the strictly moral. The authority of a code of ethics is therefore not necessarily a moral authority. A code may include legal and professional injunctions that do not have the force of morality behind them. Moral authority exists only in those elements of a code that can be given moral justification.

Regardless of terminology used, and the justification for the requirements they contain, professional codes can affect the advancement of practice by categorising some practices or procedures as either within or outside the recognised sphere of competence of the profession (e.g. injections have only recently been accepted as being within physiotherapeutic practice in the UK). Codes may also reinforce notions of professional demarcation, which may create difficulties for interprofessional working (Hewison & Sim 1998).

At a practical level, the practitioner may have difficulty in making use of a code of ethics in daily practice. First, codes are inevitably framed in very general terms, and may cater inadequately for the specific circumstances of a particular situation:

No set of rules could encompass all the subtle complexities of even the most ordinary relationship between two persons, much less the special dimensions peculiar to the medical transaction in which one person in special need seeks the assistance of another who professes to help (Pellegrino 1979, p. 51).

A second and more problematic issue is that the requirements of a code of ethics may conflict with what appears to be the ethically appropriate response in a particular case. Very few, if any, moral rules are absolute, and there will be certain situations in which it is morally justifiable to ignore a rule. For example, most codes of ethics require that confidentiality should be strictly maintained, but breaching confidentiality may sometimes, in the judgement of the practitioner, be appropriate (Sim 1996). A code of ethics does not normally cater for such exceptions, and may therefore not only fail to help, but actually impede the practitioner in acting in an ethically appropriate manner. There may be a sense, therefore, in which the generalised and inflexible nature of a code of ethics may constrain the exercise of independent moral decision-making, based on the reasoned moral judgement of the individual practitioner, and render the moral knowledge of the profession somewhat static.

Codes of ethics, therefore, face the practitioner with two fundamental difficulties. First, they provide very general guidance to action, which is often hard to apply to the specific circumstances of particular situations. Indeed, those cases that are ethically most problematic are normally those in which general rules are least useful, just as patients who are therapeutically most challenging are often those who do not fit usual clinical or diagnostic categories. Second, through the rather categorical requirements that they tend to place on professional conduct, codes can constrain ethical judgement in particular problematic instances, thereby encouraging a rather mechanical, unreflective approach to ethical decision-making (Johnstone 1994). Codes of ethics should be an adjunct to, not a substitute for, individual moral judgement in particular instances.

INDIVIDUAL PRACTICE
Imposed influences

Conflicts in practice decision-making may derive from opposing views of professional colleagues and others in multidisciplinary teamwork, or from audit strategies to show cost-effectiveness of care, or from stringent application of agreed judgements of professional codes of practice on professional behaviour. Together these influences can impose constraints on individual actions that will impact on practice development. Chief executives of health care organisations are now in positions of added authority by virtue of their role in interpreting and implementing principles of governance and managed care. Thus their performance objectives and other targets can greatly influence the principles and conditions of practice (Sausman 2001). The impact of the declared need for hard decisions to be made on 'what will we do without, to get what we really want' (Connelly 1999, p. 668) can extend from the quality of equipment purchased to the time of discharge from care (Lane 2000). In addition, requirements to promote the interests and well-being of others may increasingly be judged in the light of EBP and with due regard for public preference, as the public knowledge base becomes broader and more informed, and there is increasing acknowledgement of personal rights and of moral concern for others. Such imposed influence has implications for the development of professional practice and for professional knowledge.

Consequences for health care

An increase in the dissemination of health care knowledge, and in the regulations that surround its application, may be restrictive as well as beneficial to professional practice. The EBP movement presents a clearly defined structure that offers an attractive form of face validity for processes of decision-making in contentious contexts. However, commitment to EBP can lead to a failure to evaluate the range and quality of research upon which it is based. It is has been suggested that fewer than 50% of policy and management decisions are evidence-based (Johnstone & Lacey 2002). Today, evidence from qualitative research methods, generated from the study and interpretation of behaviours, attitudes and beliefs in specific contexts of care, may be more appropriate to the long-term management of chronic disorders and the maintenance of independent lifestyles in the community.

There are, therefore, two caveats to the idea of predicating health purchasing fully on EBP. First, the conception of EBP that currently prevails is based firmly on the standards of the randomised controlled trial and allied methods. Although these are suitable and robust means of researching the specific question of treatment effectiveness, they are inappropriate as ways of investigating certain other aspects of health care delivery. Second, even if the randomised controlled trial were to be seen as the cornerstone of EBP, there is a recognised paucity of evidence generated through this approach. In other words, not only is the current conceptualisation of EBP incomplete, but even on its own terms it has not yet provided a sufficient evidential base for rational decision-making.

A second way in which the search for greater professional knowledge may fail to further the goals of professional practice concerns the fact that research outcomes may still be more related to the individual interests of researchers and the demands of award funding bodies than to the actual needs of the professions and their clients. Furthermore, the client's voice may fail to be heard. Harsh realities of budgetary pressures, staff shortages and other managerial imperatives can displace good intentions about informing and involving patients, responding quickly and effectively to patient needs and ensuring that patients are treated in a dignified and supportive manner (Coulter 2002).

It will be increasingly pertinent to consider how harm is defined: in which health care context and by whom. For example, decisions about rehabilitation, return to work and lifestyle changes can be made in contexts of care where the vested interests of all the relevant stakeholders may mean that judgements are made from dissimilar perspectives. Legislation that protects the rights of those with work incapacity (e.g. the Americans with Disabilities Act in the USA and the Disability Discrimination Act in the UK) has done much to highlight and support individual rights to work, which can influence how health care is managed and provided, but this depends crucially upon interpretation. As Coulter (2002) suggests, there is within self-regulating professions an increasing recognition of the importance of reporting colleagues for malpractice, which may have far-reaching consequences in changing both professional practice and how the public perceives it.

With the public increasingly well-informed and involved, there is a changing perception of the relationship between aspects of modern life and health, which may exert a further pressure on the decision-making of professionals who strive to retain a profile amongst competing complementary medicine approaches. A lack of attention to conventional health advice and a preoccupation with healthy lifestyles are reflected in changes in the ways people make sense of illness and present with health complaints (Petrie & Wessely 2002), with concomitant implications for developing practice.

Implications for professional development

No one health expert can meet all the complex needs of patients and the multiple demands of contemporary health care services. Hall and Weaver (2001) point out that education in how to function in teams and how to manage conflict resolution is needed to negotiate best client-focused practice that does not compromise individual professional goals. The level at which individual practitioners are able to work in multidisciplinary teams, whilst retaining a professional distinction, will have far-reaching consequences on developing practice and on the general professional knowledge base.

DEVELOPMENT OF PROFESSIONAL KNOWLEDGE
The professional knowledge base

The knowledge base of a profession is intrinsically linked to the experiential practice of its members. In practice, clinical reasoning takes into account theoretical and clinical knowledge bases, and decision-making occurs within contextual demands. The resulting practice is based upon knowledge from a number of sources that becomes integrated through the reasoning process, and a response to a number of influences and cues in the immediate context that may sway the final decision for action. Whether consciously or unconsciously, decisions can be influenced by group preferences that are uniprofessionally or multiprofessionally dominated. The imposed structures of governance relating to resource allocation and cost implications will also make a relevant contribution. Professional knowledge is thus generated in an environment of cultural behaviour and situated action, and is an amalgam of propositional and process knowledge, personal and contextual knowledge – but, crucially, the final determining factors in decision-making reflect moral concerns. Indeed, morality may appropriately be thought of as the final filter for decisions, on the basis that a course of action that is morally suspect is not one to be adopted, whatever its epistemological credentials.

Experienced and, in particular, novice practitioners need to be aware of the combined consequences of these influences on their practice. It may be pertinent for them to consider that their individual practice at any one time reflects the body of professional knowledge upon which the essential maintenance and expansion of the knowledge base of their profession are determined.

Professional autonomy and metacognition

If professional goals are to be held sovereign amidst competing claims for practice, the act of metacognition – in which one reflects both on the essential characteristics of professional practice over a period of time and on the underpinning assumptions of professional knowledge it presupposes – becomes of primary concern as a tool to maintain autonomy of practice. Processes of metacognition offer an opportunity to abstract oneself from the daily detail and, voluntarily and consciously, to take a strategic overview of professional behaviour, clinical reasoning and clinical decision-making. The ability to recognise and regulate cognition is an essential skill for retaining autonomy in practice, and one that should feature explicitly in educational programmes (Schraw 1998, Sternberg 1998).

There is a challenge for practitioners to recognise a limit to the information and choice that can be offered to clients and to accept that ultimately interventions and lifestyles that professionals themselves see as important may be rejected. However, practitioners should be wary of seeking to make judgements on aspects of clients' lives on which they have no special expertise (Veatch 1973). Professionals can speak authoritatively on the means by which clients' goals are best attained, but not on the nature of the goals themselves (Sim 1997).

Protecting and promoting client autonomy is fundamental to a mode of practice that is in line with strategies of health promotion for client empowerment. The recent development of the *International Classification of Functioning, Disability and Health* (World Health Organization 2001), which prompts fresh scrutiny of the meaning of autonomy for individuals with disability and the balance of decision-making in their lives (Ellis 2001), is contingent upon the ability of individual professionals to facilitate client empowerment through their situated critical and conscientious decision-making. It highlights the importance of achieving professional autonomy in decision-making and reasoning that can facilitate working with change and utilising knowledge sources appropriate to the context. Ultimately, professional autonomy must be harmonised with client autonomy.

Recognising the need for change in sources and types of knowledge

The difficulties of what is expected versus what is possible in health care are becoming of more explicit concern in professional debate (Dowie 2001), with implications not only for patients but also for professions. While striving to work within traditional frameworks of professional practice, it is important to recognise the need to utilise new sources of knowledge and approaches to care. It is essential to have a clear view of professional purpose in order to be able to recognise the influences and obstacles to its fulfilment in each context. As suggested by Bellner (1999), the recent changes in views of disability and function point to an urgent need to reflect on models of relationships between professionals and clients and to realise the equal moral status of both parties in collaboration in care. Development of professional knowledge can be driven by the ways in which, and the extent to which, service users are included in care. The competing perspectives and knowledge bases of providers and users engaged in responding to the pressure for patient participation in their health care can constitute a bottom-up challenge to conventional practice. Beresford (2001), writing from a social work perspective, suggests academics and professionals have traditionally been the arbiters and interpreters of users' knowledge, and research on users' experience and knowledge has been judged, interpreted and understood by professionals rather than by users themselves. He sees the press for change in research relationships by users and their organisations, and the assertion of their moral rights to be involved in debates and developments which affect them, as highlighting the ethical and philosophical problems of not being involved. He proposes that the key moral dimension for future development of health is the extent to which users are socially constructed (Beresford 2001). The change in vision of professional practice required to embrace the full implications of shared decision-making with clients highlights a need for research topics concerned with health communication and support, rather than agendas that aim for more objective notions of clinical efficacy.

A move from provider-led and service-led practice to user-led practice underpins the moral value placed upon client autonomy. Ellis (2001) examines autonomy from the point of view of experiences of disability, showing how cultural attitudes can favour certain representations of people and can deny or ignore the experience of people who do not conform to them. People living with disabilities are vulnerable to the failure of others to recognise their authority to make decisions and to the 'situated dependence' in which they find themselves. Ellis asserts that professionals need to consider a morally acceptable notion of autonomy, which assumes a robust conception of self; she suggests that respecting autonomy may entail taking social action to deconstruct social causes of loss of autonomy and to reconstruct a society that is more enabling of relational autonomy.

Respecting the dignity and individuality of others in a multiethnic and cross-cultural context of primary care involves decision-making that may conflict strongly with professional interests. As patients become more involved with their health care, patterns of care may be set up in which accepted professional modes of practice are ignored. Over time, such practice will become the norm, and the knowledge on which it is based will predicate future development. The historical development of the professional knowledge base in response to such moral issues needs to be articulated and recorded if practitioners are to see a coherence in their contribution to health. This documenting of the evolution of the professional knowledge base should be given high prominence in education at all levels.

The importance of education programmes

It is fundamental to the development of practice and professional knowledge that students and practitioners understand the wide range of influences on their decision-making and that they recognise the moral dimensions of these influences. Although the clinical reasoning process is commonly utilised by many professions, the outcome will depend upon the focus and characteristics of the professional knowledge on which it is based. For example, a medical model may be oriented to diagnosis formulation and a therapy model may consider a broader range of categories related to dysfunction (Henley 1994). Students need preparation to distinguish the source of influences on their decision-making, so as to develop an ability to make judgements that are inclusive and deliberate, with full recognition of the reality of the context of practice at the moment and the implications for the development of the professional knowledge base for the future. The conditional reasoning component of clinical reasoning proposed by Hayes Fleming (1991), which focuses on the context of practice decisions relating to the persons involved, may now also realistically be applied to concern for the development of the professional knowledge base. Development of appropriate attitudes and orientations which create an awareness of the fluid and dynamic nature of professional knowledge can be made explicit. This is especially the case in curricula in which a situated awareness is fostered through a purposeful process of professional socialisation, one that inculcates processes of reflexivity and metacognition as intrinsic to practice behaviour.

CONCLUSION

This chapter has outlined some of the forces and processes that may influence the development of professional practice. A key question for practitioners is: to what extent should such influence be embraced or resisted? Particularly when ethical issues are at stake, practitioners need to be conscious of the responsibility of their autonomous practice which can on occasions appear to act against expected norms of behaviour, as imposed by some of the frameworks explored above. Equally, there is a need to make professional decision-making explicit, both to provide a justification for action and also to enable the evidence or insights gained to be recognised and incorporated into the professional knowledge base.

REFERENCES

Bellner, A-L. (1999). Senses of responsibility. *Scandinavian Journal of Caring Sciences*, **13**, 55–62.
Beresford, P. (2001). Social work and social care: the struggle for knowledge. *Educational Action Research*, **9**, 343–54.
Bury, T. (1998). Evidence-based healthcare explained. In *Evidence-Based Healthcare: A Practical Guide for Therapists* (T. Bury & J. M. Mead, eds) pp. 3–25. Oxford: Butterworth-Heinemann.
Charles, C. (2002). The meaning(s) of uncertainty in treatment decision-making. In *Professional Practice in Health, Education and the Creative Arts* (J. Higgs & A. Titchen, eds) pp. 62–71. Oxford: Blackwell Science.
Closs, J. S. & Lewin, B. J. P. (1998). Perceived barriers to research utilization: a survey of four therapies. *British Journal of Therapy and Rehabilitation*, **3**, 151–5.
Connelly, P. J. (1999). What will we do without to get what we really want? *Hospital Medicine*, **60**, 668–71.
Coulter, A. (2002). After Bristol: putting patients at the centre. *British Medical Journal*, **324**, 648–51.
Dougherty, C. J. (1994). Quality-adjusted life years and the ethical values of health care. *American Journal of Physical Medicine and Rehabilitation*, **73**, 61–5.
Dowie, J. (2001). Decision technologies and the independent professional: the future's challenge to learning and leadership. *Quality in Health Care*, **10**(suppl. II), ii59–63.
Edgar, A., Salek, S., Shickle, D. & Cohen, D. (1998). *The Ethical QALY: Ethical Issues in Healthcare Resource Allocation.* Haslemere: Euromed Communications.
Ellis, C. (2001). Lessons about autonomy from the experience of disability. *Social Theory and Practice*, **27**, 599–615.
Gillon, R. (1994). Preface: medical ethics and the four principles. In *Principles of Health Care Ethics* (R. Gillon & A. Lloyd, eds) pp. xxi–xxxi. Chichester: Wiley.
Hagedorn, R. (1999). *Foundations for Practice in Occupational Therapy.* Edinburgh: Churchill Livingstone.
Hall, P. & Weaver, L. (2001). Interdisciplinary education and teamwork: a long and winding road. *Medical Education*, **35**, 867–75.
Harrison, J. (1976). *Hume's Moral Epistemology.* Oxford: Clarendon Press.
Hayes Fleming, M. (1991). The therapist with the three-track mind. *American Journal of Occupational Therapy*, **45**, 1007–14.
Henley, E. C. (1994). The clinical reasoning process – how can we maximize it? *Journal of the Singapore Physiotherapy Association*, **15**, 16–21.

Hewison, A. & Sim, J. (1998). Managing interprofessional working: using codes of ethics as a foundation. *Journal of Interprofessional Care*, **12**, 309–21.

Higgs, J. & Jones, M. (2000). Clinical reasoning in the health professions. In *Clinical Reasoning in the Health Professions*, 2nd edn (J. Higgs & M. Jones, eds) pp. 3–14. Oxford: Butterworth-Heinemann.

Higgs, J. & Titchen, A. (1995). Propositional, professional and personal knowledge in clinical reasoning. In *Clinical Reasoning in the Health Professions* (J. Higgs & M. Jones, eds) pp. 129–46. Oxford: Butterworth-Heinemann.

Johnstone, M.-J. (1994). *Bioethics: A Nursing Perspective*, 2nd edn. Sydney: W. B. Saunders/Baillière Tindall.

Johnstone, P. & Lacey, P. (2002). Are decisions by purchasers in an English health district evidence-based. *Journal of Health Service Research Policy*, **7**, 166–9.

Jones, M., Jensen, G. & Edwards, I. (2000). Clinical reasoning in physiotherapy. In *Clinical Reasoning in the Health Professions*, 2nd edn (J. Higgs & M. Jones, eds) pp. 115–27. Oxford: Butterworth-Heinemann.

Kultgen, J. (1982). The ideological use of professional codes. *Business and Professional Ethics Journal*, **1**, 53–69.

Lane, L. (2000). Client-centred practice: is it compatible with early discharge hospital-at-home policies? *British Journal of Occupational Therapy*, **63**, 310–15.

Lyons, D. (1984). *Ethics and the Rule of Law*. Cambridge: Cambridge University Press.

McKenna, H. (1997). *Nursing Theories and Models*. London: Routledge.

Neuhaus, B. E. (1988). Ethical considerations in clinical reasoning: the impact of technology and cost containment. *American Journal of Occupational Therapy*, **42**, 288–94.

Pellegrino, E. D. (1979). Toward a reconstruction of medical morality: the primacy of the act of profession and the fact of illness. *Journal of Medicine and Philosophy*, **4**, 32–56.

Petrie, K. J. & Wessely, S. (2002). Modern worries, new technology and medicine. *British Medical Journal*, **324**, 690–1.

Powell, J. E. (1976). *Medicine and Politics: 1975 and After*. London: Pitman Medical.

Purtilo, R. B. (1987). Codes of ethics in physiotherapy: a retrospective view and look ahead. *Physiotherapy Practice*, **3**, 28–34.

Sackett, D. L., Gray, J., Haynes, R. & Richardson, W. (1996). Evidence based medicine: what it is and what it isn't. *British Medical Journal*, **312**, 71–2.

Sausman, C. (2001). New roles and responsibilities of NHS chief executives in relation to quality and clinical governance. *Quality in Health Care*, **10**(suppl. 2), ii13–20.

Schraw, G. (1998). Promoting general metacognitive awareness. *Instructional Science*, **26**, 113–25.

Shaw, G. B. (1946). *The Doctor's Dilemma*. Harmondsworth: Penguin.

Sim, J. (1995). Sources of knowledge in physical therapy. *Physiotherapy Theory and Practice*, **11**, 194.

Sim, J. (1996). Client confidentiality: ethical issues in occupational therapy. *British Journal of Occupational Therapy*, **59**, 56–61.

Sim, J. (1997). *Ethical Decision Making in Therapy Practice*. Oxford: Butterworth-Heinemann.

Sprent, P. (1988). *Taking Risks: The Science of Uncertainty*. Harmondsworth: Penguin.

Sternberg, R. J. (1998). Metacognition, abilities and developing expertise: what makes an expert student? *Instructional Science*, **26**, 127–40.

Turner, P. & Whitfield, T. (1999). Physiotherapists' reasons for selection of treatment techniques: a cross-national survey. *Physiotherapy Theory and Practice*, **15**, 235–46.

Veatch, R. M. (1973). Generalization of expertise. *Hastings Center Report*, **1**, 29–40.

Weiner, J., Gillam, S. & Lewis, R. (2002). Organization and financing of British primary care groups and trusts: observations through the prism of US managed care. *Journal of Health Services Research and Policy*, **7**(1), 43–50.

Williams, A. (1985). Economics of coronary artery bypass grafting. *British Medical Journal*, **281**, 326–9.

Woolgar, S. (1988). *Science: The Very Idea*. Chichester: Ellis Horwood.

World Health Organization (2001). *International Classification of Functioning, Disability and Health*. Geneva: World Health Organization.

9

Challenging evidence in evidence-based practice

Dan Stiwne and
Madeleine Abrandt Dahlgren

INTRODUCTION

Generally speaking, the aims of evidence-based practice (EBP) and evidence-based medicine (EBM) are to make clinicians more observant, more familiar with and more likely to integrate into practice contemporary relevant clinical research findings concerning aetiology, diagnosis, treatment and outcome (Muir-Gray 1997, Sackett et al 1997). When application is broadened to the field of health care, aims of cost-effectiveness and fairness are added (Birch 1997). It is assumed that much could be done to enhance the strategies and the rationality by which medical and health care are provided and carried out. Also, there is a hope that the increasing flow of research findings that emerge today will enable us to control, synthesise and evaluate its usefulness in practice. EBP thus concerns researchers, practitioners and health care providers. It is expected that a new willingness and cooperation will allow research to be informed by practice and practice to be informed by research. That is at least a two-way process, depending on how many stakeholders are involved; a process within which all parties have to learn about and take into account each other's perspectives. This is not easily done, as may be illustrated by the fact that promoters of EBM and related movements often seem to fear that the concept will be misinterpreted.

It is as if the proponents of these ideas of increasing rationality as the basis for care and treatment have ominous expectations about how the aims and goals of EBM will be interpreted and implemented. For example, Sackett et al (1997, pp. 3–4) warn that 'evidence-based medicine is not a "cook-book" medicine'; it will never result in slavish, cook-book approaches to individual care since it is a bottom-up approach that ultimately relies on clinical judgement and expertise. Further, they counsel that we should not fear that EBM 'will be hijacked by purchasers and managers to cut the costs of health care' (p. 4). And if we are afraid of a scientific tyranny over practice, we are informed that EBM is not restricted to randomised trials and meta-analyses, but 'involves tracking down the best external evidence … with which to answer our clinical questions' (p. 4). However, especially in the British debate on evidence-based health care (EBHC), the possibility of an unfair distribution of resources to patients with the best ability to benefit from care is acknowledged (Birch 1997).

Recognising that the movements of EBM, EBP and EBHC (and others with an EB- prefix) have grown amazingly quickly within no more than about 20 years, our position is to adopt a somewhat more sceptical than devoted attitude to the phenomenon. What *is* it that makes the idea of EBM so appealing? What are the strengths and the weaknesses of the ideas, taking into account that they are to be implemented by common human beings? Is the idea of evidence-based care maybe something like the ideas of 'democracy' or 'romantic love' – great ideas, but not easy to implement and to live by? How can we get the best out of EBM without being a victim of its negative potentials? These are questions that are addressed in this chapter.

The chapter starts with a description of the aims and assumptions underpinning the idea of EBM and moves forward towards questioning some of the assumptions underlying the evidence concept that is favoured by the EBM movement. We argue that research design and method should harmonise with the research questions posed, and that all research must be based on strategic choices based on access, ethics, resources, scientific rigour and generalisability, irrespective of research tradition. We also point out what seems to be a paradoxical consequence of seeking research-based, unbiased knowledge as the basis for clinical work, which is inherent in the idea of EBM. Empirical evidence of a certain health care treatment is by no means a guarantee of itself for an improvement in practice. On the contrary, we argue, it puts even more emphasis on the need for practical wisdom and the clinician's conscious judgement of each unique case.

EVIDENCE-BASED MEDICINE: THE IDEA AND ITS CONSEQUENCES

EBM aims to make medical and related fields of practice more based on empirical evidence than on tradition and experience, and to reduce variations in treatment which are not supported by sound research. It is not a question of negating what is understood as clinical expertise, but of making that expertise less based on intuition and personal preferences and more on external, scientific, systematic evidence. This is, however, far from the case today. Patients often have good reason to be somewhat doubtful as to whether the doctor does know exactly what to believe about their ailment and whether the proposed treatment is in line with the mainstream of scientific research. The following examples illustrate the problem.

Recently, at a conference on prostate cancer, persistent large variations were reported in both perceived incidence and in the recommended and implemented treatments that were carried out in different counties in Sweden. In one county only 3% of patients with a malignant prostate cancer underwent surgery, while in another county the proportion was 55%. In one county compared to another, twice as many cases were identified as malignant. This was explained by the fact that samples of tissue were judged very differently in the identification of a malignant form of cancer. The researchers suggested that the variance is due to a 'different philosophy' among clinicians as to the usefulness of identification of early incidence (Sandblom et al 1999). At a more general level, it has been reported that general practitioners and internists have a hard time deciding how to judge patients' common complaints and what to do about them. Sobel (1995), for example, showed that when patients present with any of the 14 most common symptoms prevalent in outpatient clinics, a plausible cause is proposed in less than 16% of the cases. That is not to say that physicians are generally incompetent or ill-educated, but it suggests an approach in which it is considered wise to wait and see, to reassure or to prescribe a drug that may or may not help. It also points to a knowledge gap and a need for physicians to apply new routines to obtain a more inclusive picture of illnesses, and it surely emphasises the degree to which they have to rely on their experience, intuition and clinical wisdom. Such examples could also be understood as an argument for the need for clinical practice to be based to a greater degree on systematic scientific evidence. There are numerous examples in our everyday clinical work as well as in published evidence of clinical variability and shortcomings.

It is easy to sympathise with the general aims of EBM. Clinicians need more rational, relevant and up-to-date facts as a base for sound practice. Researchers need to legitimise expensive research enterprises by their usefulness in the short or at least in the long run. Both health care providers and the agencies and institutions funding research need to be convinced that money is used for producing health. Health care providers and politicians need arguments to be able to ensure that government resources for health and medical care are used rationally. In addition, patients and their relatives have the right to believe that care is not delivered unfairly or at random with little rational base. And we all, as citizens, have the right to feel safe when we become ill. We should feel safe to trust that what is done to us as patients is founded on research, clinical expertise and experience. So far, it seems as if EBM is such a good idea that it does not need much debate or questioning.

However, there are some very important questions about the ideas and consequences of EBM that need to be considered for us to understand it fully. Some relate to the nature of the phenomena to be studied, others concern the nature of science itself. Still other questions concern those who will interpret and make use of research; that is, the practitioners, care-providers and patients. First, we will further elaborate on the scientific ideals of EBM before we broaden the perspective on the underlying assumptions, and spell out more about its philosophical foundations.

THE IDEAS OF A RESEARCH 'GOLD STANDARD' AND A HIERARCHY OF EVIDENCE

The idea of an 'evidence base' in EBM, EBP or EBHC is not only focused on what is needed, based on well-motivated ideas, in the field of practice. It also expresses clear convictions about what is *meant* by scientific evidence. Although it is recognised that scientific evidence may have different sources, the EBM movement embraces a construed and celebrated hierarchy of standards which are applied according to the design of a research study. A *hierarchy of evidence*, such as that proposed by the UK National Health Service (NHS) Centre for Reviews and Dissemination (1996) or that adopted by the Cochrane Collaboration Library (1999), is based on the degree to which a design is potent to control the independent variable and thus capable of establishing a cause–effect relationship. In this perspective the most important question to be asked, and to answer, is assumed to be: does A cause B? All other important questions regarding, for example, how the cause and effect are related, to what degree, why and under what circumstances, are seen as secondary, and relevant only if the primary question is answered as significant and affirmative. Thus, for the Cochrane Collaboration Library a hierarchy of evidence starts at the top with results derived from well-designed randomised controlled trials (RCTs) as a research 'gold standard' of evidence. Second-best evidence is acquired from controlled trials with pseudo- or no randomisation, followed by prospective cohort studies with concurrent or, second-best, historical controls. Next in the hierarchy are retrospective cohort studies with concurrent controls or case-control studies. At the bottom of the hierarchy are descriptive or qualitative studies and opinions of authorities.

As mentioned, the scientific gold standard is identified as the RCT because of its potential to give a conclusive answer to the basic question of treatment effect. The strength of the design comes from the allocation of cases at random to a treatment versus a control group and then the exposure of the treatment group to an assumed potent intervention. The control group may have no treatment, another treatment or a placebo that is not believed to be influential. Given that every step and procedure is carried out rigorously, a reliable answer to the research question will be obtained. Moving down the hierarchy of research designs there is less and less possibility to *control* the independent variable and, thus, researchers are left to *measure* or to *describe* it. The less control over the independent variable, the less possibility to ensure a causal link and the greater the risk for alternative explanations, or confounding phenomena to be accepted as valid. Note that the RCT design is, if appropriately planned and conducted, generally regarded as providing the least biased way to establish causation and to obtain the desired conclusive answer. It is also important to mention that this design makes it possible to obtain an answer that shows that a treatment is making things worse or having no effect at all. More about how RCTs should be properly conducted and carried out is described in detail elsewhere, for example by Kleijnen et al (1997) and Wessely (2001).

The EBM movement has spread to comprise not only physicians but also other members of the health care team. In nursing, it has been argued that EBM may have a negative effect on the development of nursing and health care (French 1999). The major arguments presented are, first, that EBM further medicalises the health care environment to the detriment of other perspectives that can generate fruitful knowledge for the development of the health care system as a whole. Second, the primacy of experimental research inherent in EBM inevitably defines evidence in quantitative terms, disregarding qualitative or hermeneutic forms of evidence. A final critique is that there is little known about the links that already exist between practitioners' understanding of a health care situation and the associated evidence. The need is emphasised for small-scale research projects in the practice setting, where practitioners can evaluate and validate evidence, to accomplish a more critical and informed attitude towards the clinical practice (French 1999, p. 73).

PROBLEMS AND DILEMMAS WITH THE EVIDENCE-BASED PERSPECTIVE

We now turn to three problems and dilemmas that we think are inherent in the EBM and the EBP perspective. These are the problems inherent in conducting well-controlled trials properly, in the nature of the phenomena studied and in the paradigmatic nature of the assumptions of EBM.

Problems in doing 'gold standard' research
Internal validity

As the reader may remember, the term 'properly conducted' and its equivalents are mentioned repeatedly when it comes to classifying and to making judgements about research standards. Indeed, all journals which publish articles considered to be scientific use a peer review system primarily to scrutinise the design and method used in a specific study. The question is, on what methodological arguments are the results based and the conclusions claimed to be valid? Practitioners may sometimes assume that when an article is reviewed and published, the procedure of publication is in itself a guarantee that the research is of good, if not 'gold' standard. That conclusion is, however, a mistake. When an article is published it means, first and foremost, that it has been accepted as having value to contribute to the debate about a special topic. Well conducted or not, it is considered to be a contribution to the development of research, practice or of science itself. However, all published studies are limited and biased in one way or another. This is the case because all research is built upon strategic choices concerning control, access, generalisability and costs, not least when it concerns (randomised) controlled trials. To carry out a research study, researchers have to make some important decisions about *internal validity*, that is, what is needed or preferred to restrict or screen the patient sample and control the treatment delivered and the circumstances under which the research is carried out. The question of *external validity* concerns to what degree the study is made relevant and applicable to ordinary everyday treatment circumstances. The tricky thing is that it is very difficult, not to say impossible, to have both aims fulfilled. This conflict is illustrated by the examples which follow.

Since the very idea of RCTs is to control for confounding variables or alternative explanations, the key issue is, first, to make certain that unknown or unmeasurable influencing variables are evenly distributed between the experimental and control group. However, it takes a sufficient number of patients to ensure that there are no systematic differences as to any pre-existing attributes that may affect outcome. Second, it is important to be sure that individuals allocated to the two different protocols are not selected to promote a certain result (allocation bias). Simply to state that a study is based on random allocation is not enough to ensure that selection bias is ruled out. This is because there are numerous ways in which the validity of RCTs can be compromised. One is by using a flawed allocation technique, such as coin tossing or alternate numbers. Another is to let researchers influence patient flow and allocation. Thus it has been found that bias is more readily avoided when allocation is adequately concealed, for example when it is carried out by administrators without any influence from the researchers themselves (Schultz et al 1995).

A much-celebrated form of controlled study is the *double-blind* design often used in clinical trials to study the effects of a new drug. The rationale is that, because the expectations of both patients and doctors may heavily influence the effect of a drug, both parties in a trial are blinded as to what protocol the patient is allocated. As described by Greenberg (1999, p. 301), 'medication response can be readily altered by who delivers the drug, how its properties are described, the degree of familiarity with the setting in which it is presented, and the ethnic identity or socio-economic status of the person ingesting it'. In a double-blind design, however, neither patient nor doctor knows if the patient in question is given an active or an inert drug, a placebo. This would seem to be a safe way to rule out an expectancy bias or the influence of common psychosocial factors such as hope, expectations and belief in a reassuring authority, and to ensure that an effect of a drug is truly related to its specific influence. However, it has repeatedly been shown that true blindness is very difficult to maintain. In double-blind designs it seems that, more often than not, patients are very keen to discover to which protocol they belong, and are likely to behave accordingly. It seems that they can easily detect side-effects, that is, body sensations that may result from having received an active drug. The double-blind study is thus often unmasked because the experimenter uses an inert placebo, thus seriously jeopardising the key procedure of a drug trial (Fisher & Greenberg 1997b).

This is not the place to go further into describing the pitfalls of designing an RCT. It is, however, important at this point that the reader understands that no claimed design and no research mantras like 'randomised' or 'double-blind' will by themselves make research findings indisputable.

External validity

The ambition to reduce complexity when designing a controlled study often leads to a heavy screening of patients in order to ensure that those involved in the trial have a special disease or symptoms defined by a specific protocol, and that they have no other disease or ailment that may interfere with the treatment. This is done to protect against confounding variables or alternative explanations of results. Furthermore, a treatment that is studied scientifically is often carried out under good, if not optimal conditions, by personnel who are experts and often have a strong enthusiasm and bias regarding the treatment's effect.

Now consider the following example of a controlled study. In a clinical setting the researchers encountered 130 patients who presented with a special syndrome. These were screened, to ensure they were pure cases of the type wanted for the study. As a result, 76 (58%) of the patients were considered suitable for treatment and were allocated to different protocol groups. Of these, 64 remained in treatment while 12 left the study prematurely. After treatment, 23 were considered to be fully recovered and 27 partially recovered. After a year's follow-up, 16 of those 50 relapsed, but 34 were still healthy. The data raise the question as to whether this is to be considered as a good or a poor result and whether evidence of the treatment's effectiveness is shown. Depending on how the data are looked at, the question can be answered differently. Strictly speaking, only 22% of the patients of the original selection from screening were considered healthy after a year's follow-up. If the criteria for relapse are softened to mean that the patient still had any diagnosis that was in need of treatment, then the results are still weak. This example is from a real study of treatment of depression cited by Westen and Morrison (2001) as an example of a perceived good study outcome. The standard outcome was judged as being half as good as this;

it was used by Westen and Morrison to show, among other things, that claimed treatment potential is often less well-founded than it may seem. This is because clinicians ask questions about clients commonly seen in everyday practice, and of course they ask even more eagerly about each specific case and whether a research result is applicable to him or her. Westen & Morrison introduced a new concept, 'effective efficacy', as a conservative measure of effect, to denote the likelihood that a treatment will be effective for the average patient met in clinical practice with a given symptom or disorder. This concept places the result in the context of patients *excluded* from trials and does not, as is regularly done, relate to only those patients reported as improved out of those who *completed*, or still more liberally, out of those who *entered* into treatment. For clinical purposes it is of greater interest to know about the benefits of a certain treatment applied to a normal clinical sample than to know what happened to the limited few who not only were accepted after a rigorous screening but also stayed throughout the whole treatment process.

Hence, the cardinal question concerning the results from controlled clinical trials is whether they are of relevance to common clinical practice. Does the study involve ordinary clients with ordinary complaints and ordinarily complex symptoms, or are the results applicable only to those screened and accepted for the trial? Many of the 58% selected subjects in the example above (and the proportion is considerably less in many trials) would be rarely seen in everyday practice. It is also necessary to take into account whether the treatment given is provided under normal conditions by ordinary doctors or by enthusiastic experts with a strong bias to the treatment in question.

Given the stringency of conditions, the control, the screening and all the special arrangements for carrying out RCTs and other restricted studies, we should best consider these kinds of research designs able to show a potential effect, or what can be called *efficacy*. That means that, under specially controlled conditions, with a highly screened sample, a certain treatment has shown a potential to be effective. To produce evidence from ordinary settings, with ordinary patients treated by ordinary doctors is quite another thing. Under those circumstances it may well be that results would be otherwise, although not necessarily worse. To show real *effectiveness* and not only efficacy, however, a treatment has to meet everyday and ordinary circumstances and treatment providers. Many patients are polysymptomatic, are not always compliant with recommendations, miss follow-up appointments and drop out of treatment (Holm 1993). Some take the wrong amount of medicine or take their medicine on an incorrect schedule (Stanton 1987). And in most medical treatments and procedures there is a heavy interaction between doctors and patients that has a strong effect on outcome. So a practitioner needs to look for *varied support* from research carried out from very different points of view, with both more and less control, and with both more and less relevance to practice. Looked at from that perspective, RCTs and other 'well-controlled studies' produce just one source of evidence or support, and represent studies which are intended to carry out only *one step* in an equally important continuing process of research on a specific problem. The term 'gold standard' is, we think, a misnomer that makes researchers and practitioners think that varied research designs are unimportant or of less value for practice. This impression may seriously limit the process of acquiring knowledge and may in the long run counteract the ideals that are expressed in evidence-based movements.

The nature of the phenomena studied

We come now to the more serious problems of evidence-based criteria as applied to research and practice. So far our discussion has been in terms of *process* rather than *goals*. We have pointed out that carrying out well-conducted research according to the ideals of EBM is not an easy task. That, however, is not the main issue in our effort to challenge evidence-based criteria. Every researcher can learn to conduct a trial properly, learn about the pitfalls and, if lucky, can raise funds to do interesting research. The next questions concern the goals and the implicit or tacit assumptions upon which the evidence-based movement rests. It is quite an amazing fact that the different evidence-based movements have quickly, over no more than about 20 years, won such popularity with researchers and care-providers. We suspect this has to do not only with what is declared and promised openly in basic books and articles on the subject, but also with what is hidden as implicit assumptions.

In an often-cited sentence, Sackett et al (1996), some of the founding fathers of EBM, tell us that EBM is 'the conscientious, explicit and judicious use of current best evidence in making decisions about the care of individual patients ... by integrating individual clinical expertise with the best available external clinical evidence from systematic research' (p. 71). As pointed out by, for example, Sturdee (2001), the implicit assumption is that research *can* deliver unambiguous, precise, objective evidence that is ready to be applied to practice judiciously and conscientiously. The wish for a more rational base for practice is quite understandable, but it is forgotten that the phenomena to be studied are to do with people and that it is people who should carry out the research and apply research findings in practice. Researchers in medicine wish to see themselves as natural scientists but find themselves embedded in powerful interpersonal relationships. We think that the denial of medicine as a composite of scientific ideals further strengthens the Cartesian split between body and mind and thus counteracts the ideals set up about rationality. Rationality in medicine, we think, is to accept the limits of human rationality. We believe there is an overwhelming body of research in medicine that supports the argument that scientific medicine, as it is practised, is both an art and a science and is as much human or social as it is a natural science. Medicine thus is concerned with both *res extensa*, things that have to be accepted as facts, and with *res cogitans*, matters that can be disputed or understood otherwise.

We give some examples to elucidate the importance of the non-specific or common factors in medicine. (For a more comprehensive overview see Holm 1993, Frankel 1995, Sobel 1995, Fisher & Greenberg 1997a, Scovern 1999.)

Beecher's well-known article 'The Powerful Placebo' was published in 1955. There it was claimed that non-specific or 'placebo' effects were strong and impressive within different branches of medicine. Beecher claimed that as much as 35% of placebo treatment effects, or 'satisfactory relief', could be attributed to common factors in treatments with known, precise and specific efficacy. Even if Beecher's findings have been questioned and are partly founded in somewhat flawed analyses, other studies have confirmed and even strengthened them (Roberts et al 1993).

Today, the question is not whether these non-specific but common factors are of importance in medicine or not, or whether they are limited to some special branches more vulnerable to these kinds of influence. Today, instead, there are strong indications that non-specific factors are of importance in the course of a variety of conditions, including postoperative pain, cough and headache, diabetes, heart disease, asthma and cancer. In fact, the hope of medicine to establish the therapeutic power of a drug or a treatment as a 'magic bullet' over and above the healing effects of common factors is often, in reality, impossible, since factors like hope, expectations, optimistic mindedness and belief in a personal power to promote recovery are always more or less operative. This has been beautifully elucidated by research evaluating the power of discarded treatments for different disorders and new treatments thought to be effective and introduced with great hope. Although later found ineffective, many treatments when introduced may show improvement rates of 70–80%, positive changes that last for months or even years. For example, Benson and McCallie (1979) report such effects for treatments for angina, and Roberts et al (1993) have commented similarly about many treatments such as gastric freezing for duodenal ulcers.

It is also clear today that common factors may influence the experience of pain and affect an immune response as well as having an impact on the length of hospitalisation, compliance with treatment and response to surgery (Scovern 1999). There is nothing enigmatic about these ameliorative effects. They are determined by an influential interplay between patient and doctor, where both parties are involved in shaping a collaborative partnership producing more or less expectations, hope, optimistic attitudes and compliance with the doctor's advice (Frankel 1995, Fisher & Greenberg 1997b). Thus we believe that medicine is far from a technological enterprise and should not be considered as pure natural science. The overemphasis on natural science ideals and all attempts to objectify medical practice may result in decreased patient compliance, poorer outcomes and increased costs in medicine.

In research, as pointed out by Scovern (1999), every RCT and every research placebo design is in fact a proof of the strong and important common factors in medicine. These common factors are so strong that they have to be ruled out by design, at high cost, to establish the 'pure and specific' agent that is supposed to cause an effect. Even so, in many trials the specific effect of a certain drug exceeds placebo controls by no more than, for example, 15% (in antidepressants), and for many drugs as much as 80–90% of the effect may be attributed to non-specific factors (Thase & Kupfer 1996).

The problem is that common factors such as expectancies, instilling hope and quality of the helping relationship *are* inherent in all interactions between the real patient and the real doctor. And the overall importance of the patient playing an active role in treatment and recovery is compromised, downplayed, dismissed or controlled for when described as 'placebo'. Objections can further be made that patient–doctor relationships may be and indeed have been studied by principles of evidence-based research ideas. The problem is then that two paradigms conflict. If what is known today about the patient–doctor relationship is taken seriously, and there is a really impressive body of evidence about this topic, according to Scovern (1999), then for optimising treatment outcomes in everyday practice there are good reasons to:

- maximise patient control in choice of physician
- develop third-party reimbursement schedules that reward, not discourage thoroughness and patience in the clinical examination
- preserve the physician's autonomy and status
- invite patients to be partners in the diagnostic and treatment processes
- routinely assess affect state, life stress and social support, especially in illnesses such as cancer and heart disease where the link between these factors and outcome is clear
- have physicians who believe in a treatment explain it to their patients confidently, in order to maximise patients' hope and expectation of cure.

Most of these recommendations, made on the basis of what we know about the role of common factors in medicine, complicate research and are not compatible with a view of 'natural science' for guiding practice. What is the active and precise agent in the process of instilling hope? How is it delivered and by what protocol? What is the meaning (and the cost) of letting patients choose their doctor and how do we get the time to make patients partners in and adhere to their own treatment and recovery plan? These and other similar questions show that the idea of the scientific gold standard is not applicable to many of the central questions emanating from the non-naturalistic branch of medicine. Research carried out on them must have the potential to identify its own gold standard.

It is possible to establish rigour and control in a research enterprise irrespective of the research paradigm and design. Medicine does best if it is informed by many and divergent researchers and research designs; therefore, it would be wise to downplay the ideas of scientific gold standards. It follows that the gold standard construct is a negative one for science and for practice as well. It tells us that some evidence is more valuable than others. It tells us that some researchers are more valuable than others and that some research findings are more important and should be allowed to guide practice more than others. We agree with Sturdee (2001) that overly stressing the benefits of the principles of natural science applied to medicine and related areas can do more harm than good.

Given the strong case for recognition of non-specific factors in most branches of medicine, we think it is time to consider that the science of medicine and the art of medicine are always more or less intertwined. Common factors as mediated in the patient–doctor relationship should not be seen as artefacts, as placebos or as some unethical undesired influence in care. Rather, we think it would be unethical *not* to let all factors contributing to health, well-being and recovery from an ailment be used for the benefit of the patient. We think it would be problematic to tell a patient: 'Now it seems you are well again, but the bad news is that you recovered by the wrong cause so it doesn't count and we would like to go on with our specialised treatment for a period of time'. To advocate the 'technical rationality' emphasised in the evidence-based movement may make doctors and other health care personnel think that they are doing wrong or providing something less valuable when they work to become empathetic or more helpful in instilling hope or in getting patients to be more involved in their own treatment. They may think that the most important research to carry out is to study whether doctors can make their specialised contribution in 7 minutes instead of 12 or 15. Such research may be done from a cost-effective perspective in the interest of health care providers, but it really misses the point of involving the patient in diagnosis and treatment. It risks supporting a very short-sighted and narrow perspective of effectiveness that will counteract its purposes in the long run.

The paradigmatic nature of EBM

The evidence-based movements of different branches of health care are now well established and are still growing rapidly. There are numerous journals with an EB- prefix (e.g. *Evidence Based Medicine; Evidence Based Mental Health; Evidence Based Nursing; Evidence Based Surgery*) and articles in medical and related journals with 'evidence' in the title are rapidly growing. In many countries in the western world there are now special centres, libraries or databases designed to review and to disseminate research findings to make them inform practice. The 'evidence' concept now seems to be used as a mantra that supports careers, acquiring research funding, achieving publication and a research status. We think the process is impossible to stop or to slow down in our time since it is a true expression of modernity. It assumes that the split between body and mind should go still further and that it is a good idea to further specialisation in medicine based on disease entities. We believe this trend must be challenged, modified and hampered by the insight that it represents a strong *paradigmatic* perspective (Kuhn 1962). Rather than the only way, it is but one way to look at things. A paradigm acts as a lens through which we see some things clearly but others dimly. Trapped in the paradigm, we hold some assumptions to be correct and others as incorrect. Our perspectives, which build from the paradigm, are imbued with values and attitudes. And the most important thing of all is that we don't realise that it is so. We are blinded to paradigmatic pressure and its consequences. We see no reason to scrutinise or to discuss our explicit and implicit assumptions about the phenomenon in question.

There is a growing recognition of what is called researcher *allegiance*, that is, a subtle and often unnoticed (by the researcher) bias, working in favour of the commitment of the researcher. In an often-cited recent meta-study on psychotherapy research outcome, Luborsky et al (1999) reported that the best predictor of whether a treatment would be empirically validated is whether anyone has been motivated to conduct research to validate it and whether funding committees have been ready to fund it. By carefully measuring allegiance in three different ways and comparing different therapeutic treatments, the researchers report a more than 69% variance in outcome, which is attributable to the allegiance effect. How is that to be understood? It could be that a strong commitment to a certain outcome, be it a result of a treatment or a drug or a special rehabilitation plan, makes researchers eager to find what they expect; thus, without conscious intentions, in very subtle ways, this contributes to a success in finding it. Similarly, editorial and reviewer allegiance effects have been identified (Mahoney 1978).

When it comes to the evidence-based paradigm for research and practice, Sturdee (2001) suggests that there is:

- an aim of arriving at objective knowledge
- an ideal of an impartial, disinterested seeking after truth that underpins a unified, progressive development of systematic theories, methodologies and knowledge
- conception of factual data as being value-free and independent of theory.

In our opinion, the idealistic goals and values that often go with the evidence-based movements serve more to distort a realistic perspective on research and to blind us to the shortcomings of all scientific enterprises. The key concept, evidence, tacitly claims that the person using it has some objective, value-free and maybe indisputable proof that something is or works in such and such a way. We believe there are no such proofs. At best there is some preliminary, defensible support that must be repeatedly confirmed by many varied sources. We think there is no such thing as a strict and totally value-free, impartial, disinterested seeking after truth. At best there is such an ideal to strive for, which has to be supported by a transparency about one's concerns, values and commitments. The progressive development of knowledge, then, always occurs within a special paradigm and needs the challenges of other paradigms. It is equally important to remember that knowledge is always built on data that are themselves permeated with theory and with values.

Thus, even if the evidence-based perspective is directed towards being a modern, powerful paradigm, it is still limited, in the way that all paradigms are. Research outcomes may mean many things. They do not speak for themselves; they need a qualified interpreter, a 'reflective practitioner' who is prepared to let practice be informed but absolutely not tyrannised by science (Schön 1983). Clever practitioners do best by letting themselves be informed by many kinds of evidence, be it on quantitative or qualitative bases, and by welcoming challenges from research made from other paradigmatic points of view (Buetow & Kenealy 2000). To be able to do this, we think the best way is to strengthen the professional capacity to understand and scrutinise research.

BEING PROFESSIONAL

To be professional is to try continuously to live up to the aspirations and expectations that are involved with the professional role. That means that professionals know and understand how to act and behave, socially, technically and ethically, to be able to fulfil their task. For health care workers the fundamental features of a professional role were originally outlined by Hippocrates in the Hippocratic oath (Reiser 1991) and later by Plato in his *The Republic* (Longrigg 1998). The principles may be summarised thus:

- Professionals perform within a role accepted and sustained by society. A profession is seen as valuable for society and is authorised at a certain level of capability and knowledge.
- A profession and its area of knowledge are delineated from others and the professional can understand and do things that others cannot or may not do or at least perform less well.
- A professional area of knowledge is built on scientific knowledge and the performers use a scientific language and a scientifically grounded conceptual framework.
- Professional authorised performers work at some level of autonomy, i.e. they may independently decide what to do (or not to do) within the professional speciality. However, they act within boundaries set up by rules for confidentiality and professional secrecy.
- Professionals are in contact with others and accept being members of a professional society where questions, dilemmas and the implementation of new relevant findings are continuously discussed.

Adding to these traditional professional features we would like to emphasise two more precepts:

1.   Since few medical treatments are 'magic bullets' that work irrespective of patients' cooperation, compliance or investment of hope and expectations, medical professionals are responsible for contributing to ensure optimal treatment conditions, that is, to ensure a 'patient- and treatment-friendly' milieu so as to let common or non-specific treatment factors wield their influence.

Most important, in a time when we are flooded by new research findings presented in numerous journals and books, on the internet or at numerous scientific conferences is the second precept:

2.   Professionals are responsible for their continuous updating of knowledge, for example by reading journals that synthesise and evaluate findings within their specific field of knowledge. However, research findings, single studies or synthesised meta-studies will not or cannot provide the full picture. It is up to individual health workers to add to their professionalism a more advanced evaluative competency that makes them ready to evaluate independently what the new research findings mean and how relevant they are for their practice.

Thus in this discussion we support those who see new challenges and opportunities for all health care professionals in the future. As Baker & Kleijnen (2000, p. 25) wrote:

Clinical governance will be supported by a life-long learning approach to continuous professional development and by an, as yet, undefined strengthening of regulation of the professions and their performance. For now, professional self-regulation survives but is on trial.

CONCLUSION

The position taken here is sceptical and pragmatic but not rejecting of the evidence concept of natural science applied to medicine and health care. We believe in the importance of avoiding a naive optimistic belief in the benefit of pure rationality. Sound research-informed practice could only be established through the hard work of researchers, practitioners and care-providers. Researchers must come to terms with their sometimes overly accepting belief in design and in scientific method which can solve all their problems, and they must abandon the idea that some research is less contaminated and more objective as to its capacity to rule out bias. Researchers, practitioners and care-providers alike need to understand that there is no such thing as a perfect study. All studies are in some way limited and biased, since it is not possible to take into account all circumstances and perspectives that would give a full answer to the formulated research question. To plan for and carry out research is to make choices. These choices are influenced by strategic, economic, ethical and other circumstances that restrict the possibilities to perform 'the ultimate study'. There is an inherent contradiction surrounding the validity problem in all research, that is, whether a restricted and controlled study or a study more relevant to practice is preferred. Seldom is it possible to do both. Stressing control over the effect or independent variable forces researchers to accept research circumstances that are compromised as to external or ecological validity. Focusing on making results relevant to real clinical circumstances restricts the possibilities of drawing conclusions about a real cause and opens up possibilities for confounding variables or alternative interpretations of results.

Further, researchers are human beings, embedded in social, political, economical and psychological realities. This makes them human also in their research activities, and sometimes prone to neglect results that are not wished for or are hard to publish. An urgent wish to find a treatment which is efficacious, coupled with a strong allegiance to a preferred research design or a preferred result, may make researchers unknowingly and unintentionally vulnerable to making adjustments in design and interpretations that will not do full justice to their results.

The 'cure' for the inevitable limitations in all research activities is to make professionals, care-providers and also consumers more capable of evaluating and judging what evidence is relevant and reliable for treatment. To wait for a total or even a good agreement between researchers on how to interpret results from research is often to hope for too much. To ask researchers to criticise and to present and account for all the limitations of their own research is often above the limit demanded in standards of peer reviewing, and is also too much to ask for. So a paradigmatic given will remain inherent in research and in researchers. We think, therefore, that the best way of making practice more informed by relevant research is to empower practitioners and health providers – and ultimately the consumer – to make their own judgements about research. Good research-informed practice can, however, never be established once and for all. It has to be sought continuously. It is a lifelong self-directed professional task that emphasises the important critical role of the practitioner in considering evidence from a variety of sources in the judgement and treatment of each individual case.

Lastly, and maybe of most importance, we take the ideas of EBM to mean that everything that influences medical practice in all its forms should be continuously scrutinised; not least, the very ideas of EBM and EBP themselves. Will these ideas hamper or promote practice and research development? And is there a risk, as spelled out, for example, by Sturdee (2001), that the evidence-based movement is so strong that it will attract such powerful vested interests that a debate about the ideas will no longer be a possibility? Ultimately it is an urgent task for all clinicians to execute their right to hold a personal opinion about evidence-based research ideals and to try to get the best out of the evidence-based movement while not becoming a victim of its weaknesses.

REFERENCES

Baker, M. & Kleijnen, J. (2000). The drive toward evidence-based health care. In *Evidence-Based Counselling and Psychological Therapies* (N. Rowland & S. Goss, eds) pp. 13–29. London: Routledge.

Beecher, H. K. (1955). The powerful placebo. *Journal of the American Medical Association*, **159**, 1602–6.

Benson, H. & McCallie, D. P. (1979). Angina pectoris and the placebo effect. *New England Journal of Medicine*, **300**, 1225–7.

Birch, S. (1997). As a matter of fact: evidence-based decision-making unplugged. *Health Economics*, **6**, 547–59.

Buetow, S. & Kenealy, T. (2000). Evidence-based medicine: the need for a new definition. *Journal of Evaluation of Clinical Practice*, **6**, 85–92.

Cochrane Collaboration (1999). The Cochrane Library, Update Software, Oxford. Available at http://www.cochrane.de/cc/default.html.

Fisher, S. & Greenberg, R. P. (eds) (1997a). *From Placebo to Panacea: Putting Psychiatric Drugs to Test*. New York: Wiley.

Fisher, S. & Greenberg, R. P. (1997b). The curse of the placebo: fanciful pursuit of a pure biological therapy. In *From Placebo to Panacea: Putting Psychiatric Drugs to Test* (S. Fisher & R. P. Greenberg, eds) pp. 3–56. New York: Wiley.

Frankel, R. M. (1995). Emotion and the physician–patient relationship. *Motivation and Emotion*, **19**, 163–73.

French, P. (1999). What is the evidence on evidence-based nursing? An epistemological concern. *Journal of Advanced Nursing*, **37**(3), 250–7.

Greenberg, R. P. (1999). Common psychosocial factors in psychiatric drug therapy. In *The Heart and Soul of Change: What Works in Therapy?* (M. A. Hubble, B. L. Duncan & S. D. Miller, eds) pp. 297–329. Washington, DC: American Psychological Association.

Holm, S. (1993). What is wrong with compliance? *Journal of Medical Ethics*, **19**, 108–10.

Kleijnen, J., Goetsche, P., Kunz, R., Oxman, A. & Chalmers, I. (1997). So what's so special about randomisation? In *Non-Random Reflections on Health Services Research* (A. Maynard & I. Chalmers, eds) pp. 93–106. London: British Medical Journal Publishing Group.

Kuhn, T. S. (1962). *The Structure of Scientific Revolutions*. Chicago: University of Chicago Press.

Longrigg, J. (1998). *Greek Medicine: From the Heroic to the Hellenistic Age*. New York: Routledge.

Luborsky, L., Diguer, L., Seligman, D. A. et al (1999). The researcher's own therapy allegiances: a 'wild card' in comparisons of treatment efficacy. *Clinical Psychology: Science and Practice*, **6**, 95–106.

Mahoney, M. (1978). Experimental methods and outcome evaluation. *Journal of Consulting and Clinical Psychology*, **46**, 660–72.

Muir-Gray, J. A. (1997). *Evidence Based HealthCare: How to Make Health Policy and Management Decisions*. London: Churchill Livingstone.

NHS Centre for Reviews and Dissemination (1996). *Undertaking Systematic Reviews of Research on Effectiveness: CRD Guidelines for Those Carrying Out or Commissioning Reviews*. CRD report 4. York: University of York.

Reiser, S. J. (1991). Medical ethics reflected in codes of ethics: the Hippocratic oath and the 1980 AMA code compared. *Texas Medicine*, **87**, 77–81.

Roberts, A. H., Kewman, D. G., Mercier, L. & Hovell, M. (1993). The power of non-specific effects in healing: implications for psychosocial and biological treatments. *Clinical Psychological Review*, **13**, 375–91.

Sackett, D. L., Rosenberg, W. M. C., Gray, J. A. M., Haynes, R. B. & Richardson, W. S. (1996). Evidence-based medicine: what it is and what it isn't. *British Medical Journal*, **312**(1), 71–2.

Sackett, D. L., Richardson, W. S., Rosenberg, W. M. C. & Haynes, R. B. (1997). *Evidence-Based Medicine: How to Practice and Teach EBM*. New York: Churchill Livingstone.

Sandblom, G., Mattsson, E., Nilsson, J. et al (1999). Prostate cancer registration in four Swedish regions 1996 – differences in incidence, age structure and management. *Scandinavian Journal of Urology and Nephrology*, **33**, 306–11.

Schön, D. A. (1983). *The Reflective Practitioner: How Professionals Think in Action*. New York: Basic Books.

Schultz, K., Chalmers, T., Hayes, R. & Altman, D. (1995). Empirical evidence of bias: dimensions of methodological quality associated with estimates of treatment effects in controlled trials. *Journal of the American Association*, **273**, 408–12.

Scovern, A. W. (1999). From placebo to alliance: the role of common factors in medicine. In *The Heart and Soul of Change: What Works in Therapy?* (M. A. Hubble, B. L. Duncan & S. D. Miller, eds) pp. 259–95. Washington, DC: American Psychological Association.

Sobel, D. S. (1995). Rethinking medicine: improving health outcomes with cost-effective psychosocial interventions. *Psychosomatic Medicine*, **57**, 234–44.

Stanton, A. L. (1987). Determinants of adherence to medical regimens by hypersensitive patients. *Journal of Behavioral Medicine*, **4**, 377–94.

Sturdee, P. (2001). Evidence, influence or evaluation? In *Evidence in the Psychological Therapies: A Critical Guide for Practitioners* (C. Mace, S. Moorey & B. Roberts, eds) pp. 61–79. Hove, East Sussex: Brunner-Routledge.

Thase, M. E. & Kupfer, D. J. (1996). Recent developments in the pharmacotherapy of mood disorders. *Journal of Consulting and Clinical Psychology*, **64**, 646–59.

Wessely, S. (2001). Randomised control trials: the gold standard? In *Evidence in the Psychological Therapies: A Critical Guide for Practitioners* (C. Mace, S. Moorey & B. Roberts, eds) pp. 46–60. Hove, East Sussex: Brunner-Routledge.

Westen, D. & Morrison, K. (2001). A multi-dimensional meta-analysis of treatments of depression, panic, and generalised anxiety disorder: an empirical examination of the status of empirically supported therapies. *Journal of Consulting and Clinical Psychology*, **69**, 875–99.

10

The role of practitioners in developing professional knowledge and practice

Rob Garbett

INTRODUCTION

I saw that one must oneself be a patient, and a patient among patients, that one must enter both the solitude and the community of patienthood, to have any real idea of what 'being a patient' means, to understand the immense complexity and depth of feeling, the resonances of the soul in every key – anguish, rage, courage, whatever – and the thoughts invoked, even in the simplest practical minds, because as a patient one's experience forces one to think (Sacks 1991, p. 132).

Writing when he was himself a patient after he had spent many years providing care as a physician, Oliver Sacks highlighted the importance of understanding and learning from experience. His realisation arose from a sudden and enforced change of roles that brought his new experience into sharp focus. For practitioners developing their skills and knowledge through rigorously examining their own practice, the challenge is to develop just such a freshness of vision so that they can see clearly, sometimes for the first time, the complexity of knowledge, skill and emotion that is woven into the everyday world of their practice.

In this book the term 'practice knowledge' encompasses propositional and professional craft knowledge. Other chapters (particularly Chs 4 and 6) examine research methods for the generation of propositional knowledge. Here I focus on the less travelled path of generating and testing professional craft knowledge in practice. This chapter examines processes by which practitioners can use research skills and approaches to develop their own professional craft knowledge and contribute to the body of practice knowledge as a whole. It also considers the conditions which need to be attained in order for such work to take place. By way of example the chapter draws on the Expertise in Practice project (Manley et al 2002) conducted by the Royal College of Nursing in the UK. I briefly examine the necessity for such a project from the point of view of the development of nursing as a profession before turning to the substance of the chapter – the ways practitioners can use research and development approaches to explore and extend their own practice.

Throughout the chapter I elaborate the argument that developing the knowledge and skills to examine our professional craft knowledge has both personal and professional value, as well as having the potential to improve the experience of recipients of health care. Practice knowledge has been discussed extensively both in this book and in previous publications (Eraut 1994, Higgs & Titchen 2001). None the less, if I am to set out arguments, ideas and experiences about how it may be discovered, articulated and refined I must first of all briefly outline my own understanding of the area.

WHY RESEARCH PRACTICE KNOWLEDGE?

There are compelling reasons for developing methods for researching practice knowledge. For professions, the task of developing approaches to researching practice forms part of the seeking and shaping of our identities as practitioners. Boundaries between health care workers are in a state of flux as the technology and context of health care become increasingly unstable (Annandale 1998). The search for identity and understanding can therefore be seen as becoming more contextually bound; as Higgs et al (2001, p. 4) put it, it is a time when 'rules and absolutes are replaced by radical relativity'. At the same time a range of pressures means that professionals' practice is required to be more visible than ever before, as consumerism shapes the public's attitude towards health care. But most compelling of all is the potential for systematic appreciation of clinical practice as a means for continuously improving the quality of patient care (Rolfe 1998, McCormack 2002).

The growing confidence of a range of health care professions is challenging long-enduring views of the kinds of knowledge needed by practitioners. There is no longer an unquestioning acceptance of a hierarchical relationship that privileges 'knowing that' (publicly available propositional knowledge derived through traditional research and scholarship) over 'knowing how' (the private and personal knowledge accrued through practice and experience) (Ryle 1949). This is particularly true amongst occupational groups such as nursing whose semiprofessional status has been predicated on a less discrete and formal knowledge base than that of traditional professions such as medicine.

This growing confidence has probably emerged, in part, as a response to the rapid growth of an evidence-based practice industry with its promise of rational answers to every question. Proponents of evidence-based practice themselves define it in a way that suggests that propositional evidence is not, in itself, enough:

Evidence based medicine is the conscientious, explicit and judicious use of current best evidence in making decisions about the care of individual patients. The practice of evidence based medicine means integrating individual clinical expertise with the best available external clinical evidence from systematic research (Sackett et al 1996, p. 2).

However, it can be argued that it is the 'best available evidence' that has preoccupied the majority of the academic and professional world, while the nature of clinical expertise seems to have been regarded as the unproblematic derivative or follow-on from the determination of this evidence. Is best practice simply the technical implementation of evidence-based practices? The interdependent nature of deductive and inductive forms of knowledge is largely ignored in the enthusiasm to create ever more elegant ways of predicting the efficacy of treatments (Higgs et al 2001). This way of seeing the clinical world has provoked increasing discomfort amongst practitioners, particularly in the health care professions other than medicine, where a powerful critique of the limitations of such approaches for the day-to-day realities of practice has emerged (Kitson et al 1998, Rolfe 1998, Benner 2000, SmithBattle & Diekemper 2001).

One major factor contributing to the lack of value placed on practical knowledge is the relative difficulty involved in making it explicit. The contextually bound nature of professional craft knowledge has meant that it has not been investigated or articulated with the same clarity as propositional knowledge which is created through established scientific or theoretical approaches. Yet it has been recognised that there is a rich fund of knowledge hidden within 'the guild' of various professional groups (Eraut 1994). Some doubt has been cast on the extent to which professional craft knowledge can be accessed and used. The often tacit nature or dimensions of such knowledge has been presented as a form of excuse for not making it explicit. For example, the suggestion in Benner's (1984) earlier work that there is an unknowable intuitive grasp behind practice expertise that defies description can arguably be seen as a form of elitism wherein 'experts' need not justify their actions (Rolfe 1998). Basing nursing practice on formal models and languages that can be tested and transferred with objectivity, however, may not be compatible with the ethos of nursing and with its contingent, interpretive and interpersonal nature of health care practice (Benner et al 1996, Lutzen & Tishelman 1996).

However, it is no longer either possible or desirable for practitioners to retreat to a position of not being able to talk about the knowledge behind their practice. The social and professional context within which we work has shifted to the extent where such a position is untenable. It is therefore in health care professionals' interests to demonstrate that they know what they are doing and why. Neither health care institutions (be they funded by state or commerce) nor governments or the public are willing to accept professional mystique as the justification for or illusion of quality in health care. Increasing public accountability demands have created a legitimation crisis for most professional groups (Evetts 2002). For example, doubt surrounding the efficacy of medical practice has been the source of dissatisfaction for those within and outside that profession. In both privately and public-funded health systems the realisation that medical practice, for all its claims of scientific basis, is not always supported by evidence of its efficacy has been a cause of concern (Tannebaum 1999). The origins of evidence-based medicine can therefore be seen as a bid to resist and reduce the tolerance of practice variations in health services or resources as a means of controlling expenditure and risk. This trend has flowed through to other health care professions. From within these professions and, to an extent, within medicine as well, critiques have emerged of approaches to evidence-based practice that adopt a purely technical rational approach to the use of knowledge in practice. Such approaches, it is argued, fail to consider the shifting, contextual and intractable reality of knowledge reconstruction in practice situations (Wood et al 1998).

This observation is reflected in the findings of Estabrooks' (1998) research, in which 1500 nurses were surveyed to examine the knowledge they used in practice. Nurses ranked their primary knowledge sources as experiential, institutional, medical, intuitive, traditional and, finally, literature-based. The fact that nurses in their practice do not appear to engage with research evidence to the degree that external observers would consider to be logical and reasonable (from a scientific or economic viewpoint) has been the subject of increasing research since the early 1980s.

Similar claims about the indeterminate nature of clinical knowledge have also come from within medicine. 'Clinical knowledge, including the complexities of human interaction, is not available for enquiry by means of biomedical approaches, and consequently is denied legitimacy within a scientific context', Malterud asserted (1995, p. 183). Malterud argued that three domains of clinical activity require explication: human interaction (the therapeutic potential of the practitioner–client relationship), clinical judgement and reasoning (experiential, subconscious and unarticulated processes) and a clinical philosophy (informed by values, beliefs and assumptions). This mirrors the arguments of others, for example, Higgs and Titchen (1995), who have emphasised the equal importance of experiential knowledge and formal propositional knowledge. These critiques suggest that the traditional medical model is no longer adequate to explain and predict people's experience of or needs for health care. A broader notion of health professional knowledge is required that is derived from diverse sources of reflective, tacit and interpretive knowledge as much as it is from propositional knowledge. These together can contribute to a professional knowledge base that can underpin the range of skills needed by practitioners to achieve expertise in the heterogeneous health care settings of today (Richardson 2001).

The shift of a range of non-medical professions into higher education has also created the need to be more explicit about the knowledge base underpinning the practice of these professions (Parry 2001). For nursing this has created the need to identify its own theoretical bases for practice, having historically been largely reliant on theoretical perspectives from a range of biomedical and social–scientific disciplines. It can be argued that further development of the knowledge base of health care professions requires reflection on practice and on its theoretical and epistemological underpinnings. There is a need to generate knowledge from practice that contributes to the knowledge bases of the health professions as a whole by providing knowledge claims and arguments that can be publicly critiqued, debated, refined and validated both within and outside the discipline (Titchen & Ersser 2001a).

Thus there is then a need to develop our knowledge of the processes by which the creativity and skill of practitioners are harnessed to solve individual client problems (Richardson 2001). Professionals are responsible for generating and contributing such knowledge within their sphere of work. This endeavour is important for ensuring that professionals can develop the skills to demonstrate their expertise to less experienced colleagues and students (Titchen & Ersser 2001a) as well as contributing to the development of their disciplines. At the level of patient care, it is necessary to ensure the development of well-informed practitioners, who are armed with convincing data, capable of articulating the significance of elements of their practice, and able to deal confidently with an occupational world that is far from easy (Edwards & Talbot 1994). This area of endeavour, as the production of this book attests, has been the subject of a growing literature that has sought to develop understandings of how different forms of knowledge are woven together to deliver effective practice.

THE NATURE OF PRACTICE KNOWLEDGE

It has been argued that three forms of knowledge inform practice: propositional, theoretical or scientific knowledge; professional craft knowledge; and personal knowledge (Higgs & Titchen 1995). It is the first of these that has tended to attract the most attention; however, the importance of the other two is becoming established. Indeed, not only are all three forms of knowledge equally important, they can also be used to inform and transform one another (Higgs et al 2001). For example, Titchen (2000) described in her research how theoretical principles are used in practice and are 'fine tuned' over time and transformed into practical principles through experience and through working out the day-to-day practicalities of applying theoretical and practical principles to new situations.

The term 'professional craft knowledge' was drawn from the work of Brown and McIntyre (1993); it was based on analysis of terms used to describe knowledge derived from and used in practice, and was considered to be the term that best captures the diverse and dynamic nature of knowledge derived from experience. In adopting that terminology, Titchen and Ersser

(2001b) described how the term 'craft' implies work in which performance is learned through experience and is demonstrated by practitioners who 'know their way around'. The notion of professionalism, with its inherent need to demonstrate and be accountable for standards of care, provides the context for the continuing generation, use and critique of knowledge.

However, professional craft knowledge can, at times, be difficult to access and therefore difficult to articulate and test. Titchen and Ersser (2001a) compared nursing knowledge to an iceberg, with only its tip as yet available for scrutiny and use. The challenge is to find ways in which the iceberg can be revealed. Titchen and Ersser outlined strategies for analysing professional craft knowledge, pointing out that the strategies can be applied to the needs of practitioners (regarding developing expertise and generating clinical knowledge), educators (regarding accessing and sharing craft knowledge with learners) and researchers (regarding helping them develop appropriate research methods for accessing practitioners' embedded knowledge). A range of methods has been proposed to aid the expression of such knowledge, including innovative approaches to the use of creative arts (Higgs & Titchen 2001), but their exploration is beyond the scope of this chapter.

RESEARCHING PROFESSIONAL CRAFT KNOWLEDGE IN PRACTICE SETTINGS

An important challenge facing health professionals, then, is to develop principles and processes by which practitioners, working within all the complexity and unpredictable pressures of clinical settings, can examine their practice, make sense of it and make what they find out available to others. Previous studies of the use practitioners can make of research have considered how established research methods can be employed within a workplace context. For example, Rolfe (1998) outlined how single-case experimental research, case study research and action research can be adapted and used by practitioners. Rolfe et al (2001) further refined the idea of case study research by drawing on work in reflective practice to outline approaches to reflective case studies. Although such detailed work is valuable, I would suggest that, for practitioners seeking to use research approaches for one or more of the range of purposes alluded to above, it is more important to think of the principles that need to underpin the task of examining practice knowledge. This section draws on discussions of such principles and considers the place of workplace culture in supporting practitioner research.

Practitioner research has been defined as a formal and systematic attempt made by practitioners alone, or in collaboration with others, to understand practitioners' work, with the intention of transforming self, colleagues and work contexts and developing new understandings of practitioners' work (McCormack 2002, adapted from Brooker & Macpherson 1999). There are similar themes in Rolfe's (1998) definition, in which he suggested that practitioner research refers to research undertaken by practitioners about themselves and their own practice. Practitioner-centred research, Rolfe argued, is systematic self-critical inquiry made public. It is a systematic process of generating knowledge, theory and practice, focused on itself and disseminated to a wider audience, and it is a reflexive activity that may in turn modify practice.

These definitions bear some similarity to arguments put forward for other forms of reflective activity. For example, definitions of reflective practice emphasise indepth contemplation, deconstruction and interpretation of events as the basis for learning from experience (Rolfe 1998). It is worth clarifying the distinction between such activity and research into practice. After all, reflection can be seen as formal and systematic, having a transformative purpose, being self-critical and having the potential to be made public. However, a principal difference, it has been argued, lies in the strategic intent behind these activities (McMahon 1999). Reflecting on practice may have strategic impact but its primary purpose is to ensure the quality and relevance of immediate practice. Research, on the other hand, seeks to make knowledge and theories derived from practice available for a range of possible purposes (e.g. enriching one's own or others' practice, making knowledge available to learners, providing evidence for particular practices, establishing the parameters of a particular professional group).

Titchen and Ersser (2001a) suggested that four processes are integral to strategies for exploring professional craft knowledge: articulating, sharing and critically reviewing, creating and validating. These should not be seen as sequential or entirely distinct from one another. Articulation is seen as occurring through the systematic recording of practice experience in the form of, for example, reflective diaries, clinical supervision or presentation of experiences within action learning groups (McGill & Beaty 2001). Once it has been written down or spoken, knowledge is available to be shared or critically reviewed by practitioners themselves, by colleagues or by anyone else cast in some form of helping role (e.g. facilitator, mentor). Through sharing and reviewing knowledge practitioners critique, refine and deepen their understanding of the knowledge they are extracting from practice. This in itself can be a creative act, as knowledge that is critiqued and explored is deconstructed and put together again and understood in new ways. Titchen (2000) noted the ways in which an expert developed generalisations and deepened her understanding of the practical principles that she had created, so developing theoretical principles (professional craft knowledge). Exposing emergent knowledge to public critical dialogue (and indeed to formal accreditation processes) may provide validation both locally and further afield.

A commitment to refinement and critique is important in practice-based research. As Brooker and Macpherson (1999) observed, practitioner research is a label that has been applied loosely to work that may not pass muster as research since it has not demonstrated a commitment to appropriately rigorous processes. They argued that practitioner research must explicate the following:

- the context for the research, including the origins of the inquiry, a clear statement of the purpose of the inquiry and interests of the participants
- sources of data
- the processes which transformed the data as originally recorded, through description, analysis and interpretation, into a credible account that accurately profiles the research
- well-justified suggestions about the usability or applicability of the research and future directions that are consistent with and linked to the purpose of the inquiry.

Transposing this need to demonstrate a clear audit trail of decision-making to Titchen and Ersser's (2001a) ideas, it can be argued that critique and refinement of practitioners' explorations of their practice require that this kind of detail be made available.

This level of work is demanding intellectually, academically and practically. Most health care practitioners do not have time to conduct research and may have little time to sit down and reflect on their practice (Rolfe 1998), not least because the cultures in which they work do not offer the necessary time and resources, educational or methodological preparation or the recognition that such work is necessary or useful (Rolfe et al 2001).

Practitioner research therefore needs to be situated within a broader culture that values and facilitates it (Titchen & Ersser 2001a). McCormack (2002), drawing on his own work to establish such a culture within a British health care organisation, argued that organisational support is needed to allow the principles and values underpinning practitioner research to operate in practice. This needs to be combined with an infrastructure that systematically assists practitioners to examine practice experience critically, critically review elements of practice and actively engage in experimentation in practice with a view to synthesising the learning gained. Such a culture supports individual research activities and a range of research practices, including methods of accessing evidence, coordinating research activities and ensuring ethical research practice. In other words, it supports the development of a research culture, a culture which exists to create a community of inquiring practitioners or a culture of critical inquiry. Such a culture has it roots in adult learning theory (e.g. Mezirow 1981), transformational leadership (Bass et al 1996) and theories about effective organisations (e.g. work on learning organisations by Senge 1990), as much as in the field of research. For example, Rolfe (1998) wrote about the features of the kind of critical community necessary to support practitioner inquiry. He argued that such communities need to provide an atmosphere that is:

- self-critical
- supportive
- challenging
- empowering
- non-hierarchical
- able to transcend clinical and professional boundaries
- set up to help practitioners overcome feelings of isolation
- able to locate practitioner research in the real world
- motivated to organise and empower practitioners for wider political action.

Research into professional craft knowledge, like all research, requires systematic attention to demonstrating both the processes and outcomes of inquiry. However, it needs to do this against a complex and shifting background. For this reason practice knowledge research requires support, critique and clarity of thought. The principles outlined above are now applied through a critique of a research project in which I was recently involved, where practitioners were invited to be co-researchers of their own practice as part of an exploration of nursing expertise (Manley et al 2002).

THE RCN *EXPERTISE IN PRACTICE* PROJECT

Staff at the Royal College of Nursing (RCN) Institute (UK) have been exploring the nature of nursing expertise since the late 1990s (Manley & McCormack 1997, Manley & Garbett 2000, Hardy et al 2002). This exploration culminated in the foundation of a project to support practitioners to develop a portfolio of evidence addressing the expertise they used in their clinical practice (Manley et al 2002). The project design was based on principles from Fourth Generation Evaluation (principally through a commitment to actively seeking and incorporating the views of a wide range of stakeholders in the project, for example, practitioners, service users, managers, educators, statutory bodies, professional bodies and researchers) (Guba & Lincoln 1989) and emancipatory action research (Grundy 1982) to ensure that the project developed through critique from stakeholders representing a wide range of interests.

Participants were recruited from around the UK, representing a wide range of hospital and community specialities. They were invited to take part in a variety of activities designed to help them uncover, explore and critique evidence to support their practice and, ultimately, to develop a portfolio of evidence that represented an analysis of their practice in terms of a framework of attributes of expertise (Manley & McCormack 1997). The activities in which they participated were:

- working in a 'learning group' facilitated by members of the research team, based on the principles of action learning (McGill & Beaty 2001)
- working with a critical companion (Titchen 2000, 2001) to help them collect and make sense of information about their practice knowledge
- a range of data-collection activities, including:
  - structured reflection on practice
  - 360° feedback (defined below)
  - collecting feedback from a service user
  - observation of practice (by their critical companion).

It was emphasised that, while participants were being invited to experiment with possibly unfamiliar activities, they were also being invited to take a fresh look at the evidence that they already had about their practice, for example that derived from existing professional supervision arrangements, academic work and publications.

Over a period of a year the participants compiled a portfolio, and in the action learning groups they tested the various approaches to collecting evidence about their practice supported by their critical companions. At the end of this period they submitted a portfolio of evidence in support of the expertise (i.e. efficacy, quality, relevance) of their practice, for critique by a review group drawn from their peers and from the research team. The review process was very much seen as an opportunity to pause on a continuing journey, rather than reaching an endpoint. Discussion within the review group frequently refined and clarified participants' analysis of the evidence they had gathered in their practice.

Thirty-one practitioners started out on the project. Twenty-three eventually submitted portfolios of evidence to the project team. The portfolios varied widely in volume, detail and depth of analysis. The participants carried out their inquiries very much in 'real-world' settings. Seized by an enthusiasm to explore what it was that they uniquely offered to patient care, they frequently stepped into the unknown, supported by critical companions who themselves had varying amounts of relevant experience. The paths they followed were anything but straightforward. They experienced ill health, bereavement and organisational restructuring. They changed jobs and moved between organisations. That so many of them stayed with the project is a testament to their tenacity and possibly to their recognition of the importance of developing practice knowledge and examining professional practice. The project itself generated an enormous volume of varied data. The conditions under which it was collected meant that some of it was incomplete and difficult to represent briefly. Rather than attempt to present an overview of the project as a whole I have chosen to provide a brief outline of one particular aspect of the project, the development of a qualitative approach to collecting feedback on performance from colleagues and peers (360° feedback). Within the context of this chapter, this 360° feedback can be seen as a means of generating professional craft knowledge in practice.

360° feedback

The concept of 360° feedback is increasingly used within large corporations and public sector organisations across the world. At its simplest it can be defined as 'the systematic collection and feedback of performance data on an individual or group, derived from a number of the stakeholders in their performance' (Ward 1997, p. 4). Accounts of 360° feedback describe a process in which:

- a representative stakeholder group is selected (the method for this varies from being dictated by the employer to being solely the responsibility of the employee)
- the stakeholders are asked to complete a psychometric tool (a large number of such tools can be found; for example, that of Kouzes & Posner (1995); some organisations commission tools specifically for their own use) compiled to provide feedback about the employee's performance (the employee also conducts a self-assessment)
- scores are calculated and a feedback report prepared. Depending on the size of the organisation and the amount of expertise within it, this may take place internally or through an external consultant
- feedback is provided anonymously. The literature asserts that a degree of 'safety' is afforded by this (Lepsinger & Lucia 1997, Tornow & London 1997, Ward 1997).

Assumptions underpinning 360° feedback

The 360° feedback approaches that have been reported to date in the literature have been predicated on two assumptions regarding the conditions required for acquiring and interpreting valid and reliable feedback (Lepsinger & Lucia 1997, Tornow & London 1997). The first is that feedback made anonymously is more likely to result in honest opinions about a person's performance. The second is that, in order to ensure that feedback can be aggregated and remain anonymous, an adequate number of raters need to be invited to participate in the process (usually somewhere between 9 and 30).

Adapting approaches to 360° feedback

In the project, the research team contested both these assumptions and identified practical issues such as small numbers of co-workers to provide feedback. The team developed strategies to gather feedback in a more open way, using qualitative rather than quantitative approaches. At the outset of the project participants were provided with broad guidelines for approaching the collection of 360° feedback. The processes of 360° feedback were also debated in the learning groups. This level of discussion and debate meant that the generic approach was essentially redesigned and refined through use by individuals and groups, a phenomenon entirely congruent with the project's status as a pilot study guided by action research.

Feedback on performance occurred through self-assessment and feedback collected from others. The literature on 360° feedback emphasises the importance of self-assessment. Feedback is meaningless unless it is compared with the recipient's own view. It is the degree of congruence or lack of it that will stimulate learning. To join the project the participants were asked to compile an indepth reflective self-assessment. In effect, throughout the project participants were gathering and refining their ideas about expertise through their work with critical companions and learning groups, with the result that they had an evolving sense of their own expertise which was prominent in their minds as they gathered evidence from colleagues.

At the outset it was made clear by the research team that the guiding principle for selecting stakeholders to give feedback should be the identification of people who would help participants understand their practice expertise. To draw a parallel with qualitative research, we were suggesting that participants identified a 'theoretical sample' (Silverman 2000) rather than a random sample. In other words, these colleagues were selected on the basis of first, their capacity to help project participants answer the questions being posed by the participants and their critical companions, and second, their capacity to provide the information needed for the activity at hand (Mason 1996). The range of stakeholders should include peers, junior colleagues, senior colleagues, colleagues from other disciplines and service users (Manley et al 2002). Participants were also encouraged to identify colleagues who they felt would provide both supportive and challenging feedback. In addition they were invited to consider whether their roles were multifaceted and in that case how they would obtain comprehensive feedback across the scope of their practice. Box 10.1 presents the five-step process developed by the learning groups for determining the feedback group.

Box 10.1 Steps in selecting the feedback group

1. Understanding how the workplace culture worked (e.g. issues of hierarchy and power, systems of supervision, appraisal already in place)
2. Understanding the values of those who may be involved in giving and receiving feedback
3. Finalising the format, location, timing of meetings, and who would be present
4. Identifying specific areas of practice for feedback to ensure that feedback was detailed, helpful and consistent
5. Selection of feedback group members and invitation to participate. Desirable characteristics for individual members of the feedback group were honesty, integrity, openness, breadth of vision and familiarity with the practitioner's clinical practice

Feedback mechanisms used were interviews with critical companions, feedback based on critical companion and expert participant involvement in gathering data, and data gathered using an anonymised questionnaire. Some participants received all the feedback offered to them and analysed it themselves (either on their own or with their critical companion). Others received the outcomes of analysis by their critical companions. On the whole the feedback tended to be more supportive than critical. This was a source of some frustration for project participants, as they had explicitly set out to ensure that the feedback they received would provide them with critique. However, for the expert participants even gentle challenge was enough to stimulate reflection and self-critique. A number of participants reported feeling affirmed by the nature of the feedback that they received.

By the end of the project we could argue that we had contested the positivistic assumptions underpinning 360° feedback. Through developing and testing principles underlying feedback (Box 10.1) we were able to help practitioners take the challenging step of gathering evidence about their practice from colleagues, then analysing and critiquing that evidence for themselves and finally offering their findings for further critique by their peers. Some participants were able to derive greater benefit from participation in the project than others. From the evidence we gathered we would claim that having a supportive environment in which to do such work was an important factor in enabling practitioners to develop their reflective portfolios. As indicated by the work of McCormack (2002) and Rolfe (1998) (described above), such support was not only provided by their critical companions, but was also derived from the kind of organisation in which they worked. The systematic and painstaking nature of such work was apparent. The evidence provided by the participants suggests that it was those who were able to invest most time in considering how principles could be applied to their own workplace who gained most from the process. This process was achieved through developing an understanding of the culture in which they worked and the individuals with whom they worked. These understandings were then used to underpin negotiations about how to gather data. The results were, for some, not only rich data but also improved understanding of each other's roles, values and beliefs.

CONCLUSION

This chapter has examined aspects of the role of practitioners in developing professional knowledge to underpin their own development and that of the discipline within which they work. I have argued that broader societal conditions mean that active participation by practitioners in the exploration, critique and development of the theoretical bases of practice has become a necessary aspect of professional clinical practice. Professionals can no longer rely on professional privilege or mystique to preserve their status. Rather, they must be prepared to be transparent about their practice. One response to this need has been the emergence of an evidence-based practice movement that, drawing on the precepts of traditional scientific endeavour, has sought to establish a scientific knowledge base for practice. In response, scholars arguing from more radical perspectives have suggested that the contextually bound and contestable nature of clinical knowledge is such that more discursive and responsive approaches to knowledge classification and use are also needed, if the intricacies of clinical practice are to be understood and discussed in ways that are meaningful to practitioners.

Not only must such approaches be philosophically sound, rigorous and systematic, they must also be practical if they are to be relevant and useful to practitioners. This involves attending to practice as a venue and culture to support practitioner research, as well as attending to the actual methods of practice critique and knowledge generation. The RCN *Expertise in Practice* project has been advanced as an example of how practitioners can be supported to explore their practice, expand their practice knowledge and contribute to an understanding of the nature of nursing expertise.

REFERENCES

Annandale, S. (1998). *The Sociology of Health and Medicine: A Critical Introduction*. Cambridge: Polity.

Bass, B. M., Avolio, B. J. & Atwater, L. (1996). The transformational and transactional leadership of men and women. *Applied Psychology: An International Review*, **45**(1), 5–34.

Benner, P. (1984). *From Novice to Expert: Excellence and Power in Clinical Nursing Practice*. Menlo Park, CA: Addison-Wesley.

Benner, P. (2000). The roles of embodiment, emotion and lifeworld for rationality and agency in nursing practice. *Nursing Philosophy*, **1**(1), 1–14.

Benner, P., Tanner, C. A. & Chesla, C. A. (1996). *Expertise in Nursing Practice: Caring, Clinical Judgment, and Ethics*. New York: Springer.

Brooker, R. & Macpherson, I. (1999). Communication of the processes and outcomes of practitioners research: an opportunity for self indulgence or a serious professional responsibility. *Educational Action Research*, **7**(9), 207–20.

Brown, S. & McIntyre, D. (1993). *Making Sense of Teaching*. Milton Keynes: Open University Press.

Edwards, A. & Talbot, R. (1994). *The Hard-Pressed Researcher*. London: Longman.

Eraut, M. (1994). *Developing Professional Knowledge and Competence*. London: Falmer Press.

Estabrooks, C.A. (1998). Will evidence-based nursing practice make practice perfect? *Canadian Journal of Nursing Research*, **30**(1), 15–36.

Evetts, J. (2002). New directions in state and international professional occupations: discretionary decision making and acquired regulation. *Work, Employment and Society*, **16**(2), 341–53.

Grundy, S. (1982). Three modes of action research. *Curriculum Perspectives*, **2**(3), 23–34.

Guba, E. & Lincoln, Y. (1989). *Fourth Generation Evaluation*. Newbury Park, CA: Sage.

Hardy, S., Garbett, R., Manley, K. & Titchen, A. (2002). Exploring nursing expertise: nurses talk nursing. *Nursing Inquiry*, **9**(3), 196–202.

Higgs, J. & Titchen, A. (1995). Propositional, professional and personal knowledge in clinical reasoning. In *Clinical Reasoning in the Health Professions* (J. Higgs & M. Jones, eds) pp. 129–46. Oxford: Butterworth-Heinemann.

Higgs, J. & Titchen, A. (eds) (2001). *Professional Practice in Health, Education and the Creative Arts.* Oxford: Blackwell Science.

Higgs, J., Titchen, A. & Neville, V. (2001). Professional practice and knowledge. In *Practice Knowledge and Expertise in the Health Professions* (J. Higgs & A. Titchen, eds) pp. 3–9. Oxford: Butterworth-Heinemann.

Kitson, A., Harvey, G. & McCormack, B. (1998). Enabling the implementation of evidence based practice: a conceptual framework. *Quality in Health Care*, **7**, 149–58.

Kouzes, J. & Posner, B. (1995). *The Leadership Challenge: How to Keep Getting Extraordinary Things Done in Organizations.* San Francisco: Jossey-Bass.

Lepsinger, R. & Lucia, A. D. (1997). *The Art and Science of 360-Degree Feedback.* San Francisco: Jossey-Bass Pfeiffer.

Lutzen, K. & Tishelman, C. (1996). Nursing diagnosis: a critical analysis of underlying assumptions. *International Journal of Nursing Studies*, **33**(1), 190–200.

Malterud, K. (1995). The legitimacy of clinical knowledge: towards a medical epistemology embracing the art of medicine. *Theoretical Medicine*, **16**(2), 183–98.

Manley, K. & Garbett, R. (2000). Paying Peter and Paul: reconciling concepts of expertise with competency for a clinical career structure. *Journal of Clinical Nursing*, **9**(3), 347–59.

Manley, K. & McCormack, B. (1997). *Exploring Expert Practice.* MSc nursing distance learning module. London: Royal College of Nursing.

Manley, K., Hardy, S., Garbett, R. & Titchen, A. (2002). *The Expertise in Practice Project: Final Report.* Unpublished report to Royal College of Nursing Institute, London.

Mason, J. (1996). *Qualitative Researching.* London: Sage.

McCormack, B. (2002). In search of the bull – excellence through enquiry. *All Ireland Journal of Nursing and Midwifery*, **2**(4), 36–41.

McGill, I. & Beaty, L. (2001). *Action Learning: A Guide for Professional, Management and Educational Development.* London: Kogan Page.

McMahon, T. (1999). Is reflective practice synonymous with action research? *Educational Action Research*, **7**(1), 163–8.

Mezirow, J. (1981). A critical theory of adult learning and education. *Adult Education*, **32**(1), 3–24.

Parry, A. (2001). Research and professional craft knowledge. In *Practice, Knowledge and Expertise in the Health Professions* (J. Higgs &. A. Titchen, eds) pp. 48–56. Oxford: Butterworth-Heinemann.

Richardson, B. (2001). Professionalisation and professional craft knowledge. In *Practice Knowledge and Expertise in the Health Professions* (J. Higgs & A. Titchen, eds) pp. 42–7. Oxford: Butterworth-Heinemann.

Rolfe, G. (1998). *Expanding Nursing Knowledge: Understanding and Researching Your Own Practice.* Oxford: Butterworth-Heinemann.

Rolfe, G., Freshwater, D. & Jasper, M. (2001). *Critical Reflection for Nursing and the Helping Professions: A User's Guide.* Basingstoke: Palgrave.

Ryle, G. (1949). *The Concept of Mind.* London: Hutchinson.

Sackett, D. L., Rosenberg, W. M. C., Gray, J. A. M., Haynes, R. D. & Richardson, W. S. (1996). Evidence based medicine: what it is and what it isn't. *British Medical Journal*, **312**(1), 71–2.

Sacks, O. (1991). *A Leg to Stand On.* London: Picador.

Senge, P. (1990). *The Fifth Discipline: The Art and Practice of the Learning Organization.* London: Century Business.

Silverman, D. (2000). *Doing Qualitative Research: A Practical Handbook.* London: Sage.

SmithBattle, L. & Diekemper, M. (2001). Promoting clinical practice knowledge in an age of taxonomies and protocols. *Public Health Nursing*, **18**(6), 401–8.

Tannebaum, S. J. (1999). Evidence and expertise: the challenge of the outcomes movement to medical professionalism. *Academic Medicine*, **74**(7), 757–63.

Titchen, A. (2000). *Professional Craft Knowledge in Patient-Centred Nursing and the Facilitation of its Development.* University of Oxford DPhil thesis. Oxford: Ashdale Press.

Titchen, A. (2001). Critical companionship: a conceptual framework for developing expertise. In *Practice Knowledge and Expertise in the Health Professions* (J. Higgs & A. Titchen, eds) pp. 80–90. Oxford: Butterworth-Heinemann.

Titchen, A. & Ersser, S. (2001a). Explicating, creating and validating professional craft knowledge. In *Practice Knowledge and Expertise in the Health Professions* (J. Higgs & A. Titchen, eds) pp. 48–56. Oxford: Butterworth-Heinemann.

Titchen, A. & Ersser, S. (2001b). The nature of professional craft knowledge. In *Practice Knowledge and Expertise in the Health Professions* (J. Higgs & A. Titchen, eds) pp. 35–41. Oxford: Butterworth-Heinemann.

Tornow, W. W. & London, M. (1997). *Maximizing the Value of 360-Degree Feedback.* San Francisco: Jossey-Bass.

Ward, P. (1997). *360 Degree Feedback.* London: Institute of Personnel and Development.

Wood, M., Ferlie, E. & Fitzgerald, L. (1998). Achieving clinical behaviour change: a case of becoming indeterminate. *Social Science and Medicine,* **47**(11), 1729–38.

11

Clinical reasoning and practice knowledge

Joy Higgs, Mark Jones, Ian Edwards and Sarah Beeston

INTRODUCTION

Clinical reasoning (or clinical decision-making) provides a bridge between practice and knowledge; it can be thought of as the use of knowledge in practice and it provides a means for generating and refining knowledge through practice. In this way, clinical reasoning provides a vehicle for practice epistemology to be manifest within practice. Practice knowledge can be critiqued and extended through the heightened awareness that clinical reasoning (or knowing-in-action) requires. This awareness enables practitioners to identify limitations of their current knowledge and recognise emerging clinical patterns which are precursors to knowledge generation. This chapter presents clinical reasoning as the core of professional practice and a key dimension in expertise and in professional development. In particular, clinical reasoning is the process which can enable relevant and emerging practice knowledge to be utilised appropriately. In the process of clinical reasoning, knowledge is critiqued and utilised within the current clinical task, but it is also evaluated in relation to a longer-term perspective which prompts the revision and continued generation of knowledge.

To be competent, practitioners need to be able to draw on the variety of practice knowledges explored throughout this book (especially Chs 3, 4 and 6) and to critique and integrate them through clinical reasoning to make sound clinical decisions and take action relevant to the setting and client. Expert practitioners learn to generate, critique and use knowledge with considerable finesse; this has been called judgement artistry (Paterson & Higgs 2001). In this chapter we examine the role of clinical reasoning in competent and expert practitioners engaged in clinical reasoning, including ethical and collaborative decision-making. We look at the way clinical reasoning can utilise knowledge from many sources (practice, research, theory, experience) to achieve these ends; and the way clinical reasoning provides a powerful vehicle for knowledge generation and professional development.

To address these issues the chapter deals with the following topics:

- understanding the nature of clinical reasoning and the process of clinical reasoning as the use of practice knowledge in practice
- the links between clinical reasoning, expertise, judgement artistry and practice knowledge
- clinical reasoning as a vehicle for generating, critiquing and refining the practice knowledge base of practitioners and their professions.

UNDERSTANDING CLINICAL REASONING AS THE USE OF PRACTICE KNOWLEDGE IN PRACTICE

Clinical reasoning refers to the thinking and decision-making processes which occur in professional practice. In some professions the context of this decision-making is clearly clinical, implying direct patient or client care in a health care context. For others the context is non-clinical (e.g. industry, schools, community settings), and the professional practice may be oriented to groups and to health promotion rather than individual health care. Most of the literature examining clinical reasoning (and professional decision-making) refers to the clinical context. We ask our readers to translate this as applicable to their work settings.

Research into clinical reasoning demonstrates an early emphasis on the cognitive processes of reasoning and a growing recognition that clinical reasoning involves an integral link between cognition, metacognition (or reflective self-awareness) and practice knowledge (Higgs & Jones 2000). Research-based understanding of clinical reasoning has evolved considerably from its origins in medical education research with its mission of helping to teach physicians how to diagnose accurately and efficiently. An enduring clinical reasoning model in medicine, which was derived from the cognitive science perspective, is the hypothetico-deductive method or hypothesis generation and testing (Elstein et al 1978). Early models of clinical reasoning in nursing and allied health reflected this inheritance from medical research (Rogers & Masagatani 1982, Payton 1985, Jones 1988).

More recently, explanations of clinical reasoning have also taken account of the organisation and accessibility of practice knowledge stored in the clinician's memory, not just the process of reasoning. Examples of such clinical reasoning models include 'illness scripts' (Schmidt et al 1992) and 'pattern recognition' (Patel & Groen 1986). With illness scripts or pattern recognition there is an instantaneous recognition by clinicians of particular features of a case. This recognition activates other relevant information in the clinician's stored network of practice knowledge, including 'if–then' rules of production, such as likely treatment regimes and contraindications (Arocha et al 1993). With the use of pattern recognition or illness scripts, clinicians move in their thinking from a set of specific observations toward a generalisation, so it is known as forward reasoning (Patel & Groen 1986). Forward reasoning contrasts with hypothetico-deductive reasoning in that the latter moves from a generalisation (multiple hypotheses) towards a specific conclusion (e.g. diagnosis). Hypothetico-deductive reasoning is used by more inexperienced practitioners but it also occurs in situations where experts are faced with an unfamiliar problem or more complex presentation. Pattern recognition is faster and more efficient and is used by expert and experienced practitioners in their domain (Patel & Groen 1986). The link between the accumulation of practice knowledge through learning and experience and the capacity to perform expert processes of reasoning begins to emerge in the pattern recognition model of clinical reasoning.

The models of clinical reasoning described above are widely accepted in medicine and have their basis in an empirico-analytical or scientific research paradigm. Diverging from this paradigm, researchers in allied health, particularly nursing, occupational therapy and later physiotherapy began to research the development of clinical expertise and clinical reasoning of health practitioners away from the laboratory and at the site of clinical practice (e.g. Mattingly & Hayes Fleming 1994, Benner et al 1996, Jensen et al 1999). On the whole, this research adopted an interpretive research paradigm approach which could take account of and value the many variables found in clinical practice over which a researcher would have little control.

As a result of this research, several models or explanations of clinical reasoning have been proposed. The main models are *intuitive reasoning* (Benner & Tanner 1987), *narrative reasoning* (Mattingly 1991), *interactive reasoning* and *conditional reasoning* (Fleming 1991), *practical reasoning* (Jensen et al 1999), *pragmatic reasoning* (Schell & Cervero 1993), *predictive reasoning* (Hagedorn 1996) and *ethical reasoning* (Gordon et al 1994). These newer conceptions of clinical reasoning in allied health have broadened the traditional concept of clinical reasoning as being concerned mainly with diagnosis. Rather than a primarily unilateral cognitive process occurring within the head of the practitioner, clinical reasoning has come to be understood as an interactive process between clinician and client (and carers/family), as many of the models of interactive reasoning reflect. In addition to diagnostic decisions about the cause of disease or disability, there is also an imperative in these newer models of reasoning to understanding clients' (and/or carers') experiences of illness or disability (Mattingly 1991). Thus, recent literature regarding clinical reasoning and clinical expertise emphasises aspects of clinical practice beyond the strictly biomedical, such as interaction, collaboration, teaching and caring practice (Benner et al 1996, Gastmans et al 1998, Jensen et al 1999, Jones et al 2000). As a result of this expansion in the modelling of the nature of clinical reasoning, practice knowledge in its various forms (including experience-based knowledge) became more clearly identified as vital to the reasoning process. Increasingly, the place of professional craft knowledge in reasoning (e.g. knowledge of how to deal with people in their unique situations) can be seen to play an important role in reasoning, particularly in collaborative reasoning.

A recent example of such research is that of Edwards (2001), who used an interpretive methodology to study the clinical reasoning of physiotherapists in three different fields of physiotherapy: musculoskeletal, neurological and domiciliary care. He observed that the therapists in each of the three fields consistently attended (in terms of foci of thinking and action) to a wide range of activities in clinical practice. These foci of thinking and action were termed *clinical reasoning strategies* and included:

- formation of diagnosis (diagnostic reasoning)
- understanding clients and their context (narrative reasoning)
- determination of and carrying out treatment procedures (reasoning about procedure)
- establishing and managing the therapist–client relationship (interactive reasoning)
- nurturing a collaborative approach towards deciding and implementing goals of treatment (collaborative reasoning)
- engaging in individualised and context-sensitive teaching (reasoning about teaching)
- envisioning future scenarios with clients and exploring their choices and their implications (predictive reasoning)
- apprehension and resolution of ethical and pragmatic dilemmas (ethical reasoning).

The current understanding of clinical reasoning as a client-centred process which integrates the many complex functions and activities of clinical practice has several characteristics (Higgs & Jones 2000). First, the practitioner utilises three core elements in reasoning: (1) cognition or reflective inquiry, where thinking skills are used to process data; (2) a strong, discipline-specific, multidimensional practice knowledge base; and (3) metacognition. Metacognition provides the integrative element between cognition and practice knowledge. It assists practitioners to uncover links or inconsistencies between clinical data and expectations based on prior learning, and allows the practitioner to examine the assumptions underlying decision-making. Second, the practitioner reasons within the context of the client's situation and task. Contextual interaction involves interactivity in the reasoning process between the decision-makers and the personal circumstances, situation or physical home and work environment of clients. Reasoning, therefore, needs to involve a consideration of the impact of the clinical task (its nature, uniqueness, changeability and multidimensionality) on the reasoning process. Finally, the reasoning process, wherever possible, should involve mutual decision-making, whereby the decision-making role of the client or patient is facilitated and nurtured by practitioners.

Engaging with people (clients, carers, family, other professionals) during clinical reasoning and clinical practice demands the capacity to behave ethically and collaboratively. Ethics in health care is an extensive field. While health care practitioners are regularly faced with ethical and moral decisions, many have received little theoretical preparation or practical guidance for resolving the wide spectrum of ethical dilemmas they encounter in practice. Like other areas of decision-making, ethical decision-making is often tacit, involving judgements and actions learned through individual experiences without explicit awareness of the salient cues and associated reasoning underpinning the decisions made. In fact, debate within the ethics literature wrestles with this very issue; that is, to what extent should ethical decisions be based on set rules (for example, as constructed by broad principles set out by a professional body, with the notion that what is 'good' or 'right' can be universally applied), and to what extent should these decisions be informed by narratives of previous ethical dilemmas, where the context of the situation, as much as any broader rule of right and wrong, guides decisions and actions? Here we take the stance that, as in other areas of decision-making, competent practitioners should be guided by a combination of community and professional standards (propositional knowledge) adopted in a context-sensitive manner as learned through previous experiences (i.e. using professional craft knowledge). We are here in accordance with Benner (1991, p. 18), who wrote:

Ethics in health care must start with practice-based understanding of what it is to be a person, what constitutes the relationships among the health care worker, patient, family, and community, and what constitutes care and responsibility toward one another.

The scope of ethical decisions facing health care practitioners can range from issues of life and death to more commonplace, yet important, decisions of client autonomy, informed consent, confidentiality, interprofessional relationships, practitioner–client relationships, resource distribution/cost containment and the myriad of day-to-day decisions that underpin quality care. Clinical decisions that are based solely on the practitioner's judgement of what is best for the client are not consistent with ethical decision-making, which inherently recognises that decisions made for the client need to be made with the client, wherever possible. For clinical decisions to be ethical decisions, and for the practitioner to provide health care that is truly caring, there is a need for awareness of and sensitivity to clients' circumstances and to the meanings they (and their significant others) attach to their illness or disability. That is, while broad principles of biomedical ethics provide a useful structure by which to orient practitioners to ethical issues, the ethical decisions themselves must be made within the context of each client's illness experience (Mattingly 1991). In this sense, ethical reasoning needs to be informed by narrative reasoning, in which biopsychosocial knowledge alone is insufficient and must be augmented by knowledge derived from experience, including professional craft and personal knowledge. Such experience-based knowledge enables practitioners to understand the person behind the problem, to discover how the problem impacts on the person's life, and how the person is or is not coping; and to do all of this with sensitivity, respect and empathy (White 2001).

Understanding the client's perspective, including the bases of that perspective, is essential to making ethical decisions. Decisions regarding the client's meaning perspective and illness experience, by their very nature, cannot be reduced to simple biomedical principles or universal truths. Likewise, ethical decision-making cannot always consist of the application of an established bioethical principle to a given situation or dilemma (Benner 1991, Nicholas & Gillett 1997). Ethical judgements require in the first instance a consensus between practitioner and client regarding their actual perspectives or experiences. It is optimal for practitioners to have insight not only into the assumptions and values underlying their clients' views or decisions, but also into the assumptions and values underlying their own attitudes, and an understanding of how decisions in clinical practice can uncover or give rise to ethical dilemmas (Barnitt 1998). Such attitudes and values are shaped for the health practitioner in part by ethical principles learned or refined during professional socialisation and in part by personal knowledge and experiences. Ethical decision-making necessarily occurs within a clinical reasoning framework formed by a sound knowledge of the code of conduct and ethical principles of the relevant profession and an ability to understand the unique features and experiences which give rise to the particular dilemma facing client and practitioner.

Collaborative reasoning is intrinsically related to an ethical principle of client autonomy (Sim 1998) and to humanistic principles underlying the caring professions. Like ethical decision-making, collaborative reasoning builds on an understanding of the unique qualities and characteristics of clients, their problems or disabilities and the context in which they exist. Collaborative reasoning recognises that there is a clinical reasoning process occurring not only within the practitioner but also within the client (Edwards 2001). In other words, if practitioners are forming hypotheses regarding clients' problems with a view to instituting clinical action, it is important to realise that clients are also forming (or have formed) hypotheses regarding their health problems, the potential causes of these problems and their likely implications for their lives. Practitioners' interpretations of problems may not be neutral in their effects on clients' symptoms or disabilities and may, in turn, have profound effects on clinical decision-making, possibly for the worse (White & Epston 1990). That is, clients' beliefs about their symptoms or disabilities may cause them to make responses or take actions which further contribute to their problem. For example, the belief that any activity which leads to back pain will necessarily cause further damage can result in several outcomes which, paradoxically, appear to confirm the reasoning of the client: as the client does less and hence gradually becomes more physically deconditioned and less confident, more and more activities of daily living will cause back pain. The client's beliefs concerning the relationship between activity and damage are thus strengthened. However, it is obvious that this reasoning is not necessarily sound. Readers may be able to cite similar examples of distorted reasoning from their own fields of practice.

The task of practitioners when engaging in collaborative reasoning is, first, to create a coherence between these two reasoning processes (theirs and that of the client) by generating a common space between themselves and the client in which the assumptions behind the actions or decisions of either party can be questioned and evaluated. Reasoning in this manner has strong links to a process of adult learning which is aimed at transformation of existing perspectives (Mezirow 1991). Again, it can apply to either practitioner or client. Effective collaborative reasoning means that there is great potential for both to learn from the clinical encounter. Edwards (2001) found that expert physiotherapists in different fields of physiotherapy practice were unanimous in the high value they placed on what they learned from their clients in clinical practice. Some of the knowledge which these therapists valued was clinically useful for similar future situations; at other times it impacted in a personal way on therapists' professional and personal values and their understandings of their own practices. To this extent, collaborative decision-making was regarded by these therapists as not only indispensable to effective practice but often practice-enriching.

Collaborative reasoning has the following strands: effective communication across perspectives, a process of evaluation (or negotiation) and new learning on the part of the protagonists. In terms of health care practitioners, the new learning may be made up of different types of propositional, professional or personal knowledge which then feed back into their practices and the development of expertise (Benner et al 1996, Jensen et al 1999). It is not surprising, then, that there is increasing evidence that collaborative decision-making leads to improved outcomes in health care (Lorig et al 1999, Radovich 2001).

THE LINKS BETWEEN CLINICAL REASONING, EXPERTISE, JUDGEMENT, ARTISTRY AND PRACTICE KNOWLEDGE
Clinical reasoning and practice knowledge

There are many ways of understanding the connection between practice knowledge and clinical reasoning: their interdependence in action, the importance of discipline-specific and generalised knowledge in reasoning, the value of knowledge structures and categorisations and the nature of the knowledge base in experts. According to Nickerson et al (1985), knowledge and thinking are interdependent, since the development of knowledge requires thinking, and thinking can be defined as the ability to apply knowledge. The importance of discipline- or domain-specific knowledge in professional decision-making and problem-solving expertise is widely stressed (Grant & Marsden 1987). Glaser and Chi (1988) found that experts excel in their own domains, using large meaningful patterns of knowledge to solve problems. Yet even such extensive, rich knowledge bases are insufficient for sound clinical reasoning to occur. As well as relevant knowledge, skills in cognition and metacognition are essential for effective thinking and problem-solving (Alexander & Judy 1988). Cognition includes thinking which is critical, creative, reflective and dialectical (i.e. coping with competing/multiple interests) (Basseches 1984).

The growing recognition in clinical reasoning research of the importance of practice knowledge within the reasoning process has been paralleled by a growth in exploration of the various forms of knowledge used in health professional practice. In Chapter 4, forms of knowledge are discussed and four key forms of knowledge which have value in professional practice are identified:

1. propositional knowledge (which describes and predicts)
2. procedural knowledge (which enables action)
3. theoretical knowledge (which explains and interprets)
4. emancipatory knowledge (which empowers people).

In clinical practice, these four forms of knowledge are used to address the imprecise (grey) areas of practice and to appreciate the many human dimensions of health care. Clinicians who adopt a client-centred approach will need to explore both the illness and the life experiences of their clients. Each of these knowledge forms contributes to the finding of the 'common ground' between client and clinician, which is seen by Stewart and Brown (2001) as necessary in three key areas:

1. identifying the nature of the problem
2. negotiating the goals of treatment or management
3. clarifying the roles of both the clinician and the patient or client.

They further suggest that clinicians and patients (or clients) have widely divergent views in each of these areas, views which need to be taken into consideration during collaborative reasoning.

Restricting ourselves to any single form of knowledge or way of knowing can result in a limitation of the range of knowledge and the depth of understanding available within a given problem situation. Health professionals rely upon the scientific knowledge of human behaviour and body responses in health and illness, the aesthetic perception of significant human experiences, a personal understanding of the uniqueness of the self and others, and the ability to make decisions within concrete situations involving particular moral judgements. Each of these ways of knowing has a place in the practice of clinical reasoning. Propositional knowledge is derived through research and/or scholarship, is formal, explicit and exists in the public domain; it facilitates the analysis of clients' psychosocial and physical problems. Using professional craft knowledge (derived from professional experience) the clinician can integrate different forms of clinical data and place physical and psychosocial assessment findings within the context of the client's unique needs (Rew & Barrow 1987). This knowledge enables clinicians to make procedural decisions such as selecting and timing data collection, in order to consolidate their understanding of the particular clinical problem (Jensen et al 1992). As well as domain-specific knowledge, clinicians need personal knowledge gained from their life experience. Personal knowledge provides a uniquely individualised form of knowledge invaluable in facilitating interpersonal interactions that are necessary for client-centred care.

Practice knowledge arising from research as well as from practice experiences is essential to clinical decision-making. Research knowledge can be categorised according to the research paradigm from which it derives, and these paradigms provide a rich variety of knowledge to inform and enrich practice. Knowledge from the empirico-analytical paradigm provides clinicians with the domain-specific scientific and theoretical knowledge necessary for identifying the nature of their clients' problems. Common presenting problems are classified through experimental research; outcome studies provide some indication of time-scales for recovery; clinical research offers examples of solutions that have been effective in relation to given clinical problems. Knowledge from this paradigm is particularly useful in dealing with the physical domain, as it informs diagnostic and prognostic thinking. However, for the most part this knowledge is not accessible to clients, who may have a quite different view of the nature of their problems (even with the growing access of the public to medical knowledge via the internet).

If clinicians are to understand the conceptions held by their clients, they need to understand something of their illness experiences and life circumstances. Such understanding draws on the more descriptive knowledge offered by the interpretive research paradigm, which focuses on human phenomena and portrays problems and people in their natural contexts. The increasing number of phenomenological studies within nursing and other branches of health care provide insight into the lived experience of patients and clients. These can enhance clinicians' appreciation of what is entailed in living with, for example, chronic pain (O'Loughlin 1999) or breathlessness (Nicholls 2000). Clinicians are helped to reconceptualise the nature of their clients' problems, taking account of their illness experience as well as their disease process. This paves the way for negotiating mutually acceptable goals that incorporate the values and priorities of both parties. The very principle of client-centred care requires a sharing of knowledge and a mutual agreement of proposed plans and actions, respecting the values of all concerned.

The process of negotiation and agreement that is inherent in clinical decision-making is informed by ethical guidelines and understanding of sociocultural dynamics that are pertinent to ways in which health care professionals and clients work together. The critical research paradigm gives rise to such ethical, social and emancipatory knowledge. In both research and practice, critical debate within professions has led to the development of codes of practice and principles of good/best practice. However, negotiations are unlikely to be effective unless clinicians appreciate the dimensions of clients' illness experiences, such as:

- their feelings, especially their fears about being ill
- their ideas about what is wrong with them and the basis of those ideas
- the impact of their problems on their lives
- their expectations about what should be done
- their sense of agency or powerlessness.

The fourth knowledge generation framework we present here is the creative arts paradigm. Research and theorising in this paradigm can produce propositional knowledge related to aesthetic dimensions of life and practice. In addition, the creative arts offer a means of generating experience-based knowledge such as embodied, spiritual and intuitive knowledge. Such knowing helps clinicians to appreciate more deeply the client's situation, to see the whole person and sense the potential of the individual when participating as a partner in managing the problem.

Clinical expertise and practice knowledge

Clinical expertise is not an endpoint but a journey; it can be viewed as a continuum along multiple dimensions, including effectiveness and appropriateness of clinical outcomes, professional judgement, technical clinical skills, communication and interpersonal skills, a sound knowledge base, and cognitive and metacognitive proficiency (Higgs & Jones 2000). Research has demonstrated that experienced and expert practitioners use practice knowledge differently (i.e. in a more integrated way), that their knowledge bases are richer and deeper than those of novices (hence their greater capacity for pattern recognition, as discussed above), that their knowledge becomes more organised and integrated with practice (Schmidt & Boshuizen 1993), and that they rely more on clinical, experience-based knowledge than biomedical, propositional knowledge (Boshuizen & Schmidt 2000). In addition, Eraut

(1994) and Titchen (2000) have contended that experienced practitioners transform theory in a variety of ways in order to make it useful to individual clients in their unique situations. The capacity to provide personalised care is a key element of expertise that develops from clinical practice experience (Benner 1984, Burke & DePoy 1991, Jensen et al 1992).

The ability to assess the importance of information and detect and interpret crucial cues has been found to arise from the capacity of experienced professionals to integrate propositional knowledge with professional craft knowledge (Dreyfus & Dreyfus 1986, Elstein et al 1990). The integration of both forms of knowledge into 'well-developed and easily accessible schemata … [enables practitioners] to evaluate and treat different patients efficiently and with confidence' (Jensen et al 1992, p. 718). Effective professional practice relies on the interdependency (often ignored in evidence-based practice discourse) between theoretical knowledge and knowledge from professional practice experience, both of which are embedded in the context of professional practice. Professional practice without underpinning theory lacks substantiation. Utilising theory in practice without considering the practice context may result in ineffective treatment and management decisions, or decisions considered irrelevant by the client. Mere application (which can often be uncritical and generalised) of theory or research findings may be indicative of inexperience. Clinical reasoning provides the means of examining the relevance of knowledge to specific practice situations.

In a broad study of experts, Glaser and Chi (1988) identified a number of characteristics that pertain to the use of practice knowledge in clinical reasoning, including the ability to perceive large meaningful patterns in the domain, to see and represent a problem in the domain at a deeper (more principled) level than novices, to solve problems quickly with little error, to demonstrate superior short-term and long-term memory, and to utilise strong self-monitoring skills. Within today's customer-focused world of clinical practice we should be able to expect that experts not only achieve successful outcomes and technical excellence but also engage in client-centred practice (including collaborative decision-making), that they can articulate and justify their reasoning (recognising the cultural and knowledge backgrounds of their audience, whether clients or colleague) and draw on the rich resources of a variety of practice knowledge, using this knowledge critically (Higgs & Jones 2000).

If we examine these expert characteristics (and expectations), the issue of practice epistemology is clearly relevant. To achieve higher levels of performance, such as expertise, practitioners need to know about and be able to use knowledge that is relevant to their practice, to know how to use a range of knowledge in their practice and to do so, to monitor this knowledge use (metacognitively, critically, reflexively), to value the knowledge of others and be able to create as well as refine knowledge.

The link between knowledge use/growth and expertise is central to a model of expertise development in medicine produced by Schmidt and Boshuizen (1993). This model presents four stages of expertise development, described largely in terms of how knowledge, cognitive structures and memory are used in relation to clinical practice:

- In Stage 1, medical students develop elaborate networks of pathophysiological knowledge which they use to explain the causes or consequences of disease.
- In Stage 2 these elaborate explanations are truncated into more clinically based explanations of signs and symptoms. Concept clusters are formed as students repeatedly identify direct lines of reasoning between clinical presentations and diagnostic categories and explanations.
- In Stage 3, continued clinical experience and increasing exposure to clinical situations result in further knowledge transformation. The existing networks of knowledge are transformed into *illness scripts* (a means of cognitively storing information for subsequent use). Illness scripts are activated as further encounters with clinical cases occur; they guide the clinician through the examination and diagnostic process.
- In Stage 4, as clinicians develop more and more illness scripts, these scripts are transformed from rather general information structures into more 'instantiated' or specific example scripts in which expert physicians are able to recall the details of individual clients' clinical presentations many years after the encounter. In this way the increasing organisation of clinical knowledge and experience stored in the memories of experts can be explained, and expertise in rapid and accurate diagnosis can be interpreted as a form of pattern-matching with former similar clients.

This model of clinical expertise development highlights two significant points in relation to clinical reasoning and practice knowledge. The first is that expertise needs to be seen not just as a measure of outcome effectiveness or achievement, but also as a measure of the capacity for and demonstration of sound clinical reasoning. The second is that growing competence in clinical reasoning as a characteristic of emerging expertise is inextricably linked to the expansion and greater organisation and networking of the practitioner's knowledge base progressively to encompass an increasing proportion of clinical experience-based knowledge.

One of the challenges facing practitioners today is to learn to value the different forms of knowledge highlighted in Schmidt and Boshuizen's (1993) stage model of expertise. The model recognises the important place of clinical, experience-based knowledge, particularly instantiated or patient-specific knowledge (along with research and biomedical knowledge) in expert practice. By comparison, the evidence-based practice movement emphasises research knowledge of a generalised (population-relevant) nature.

Evidence-based practice involves basing clinical decisions and practice on the best available evidence. Sackett et al (2000, p. 1) described evidence-based medicine as 'the integration of best research evidence with clinical expertise and patient values'. These authors defined best research evidence as 'clinically relevant research, often from the basic sciences of medicine, but especially from client-centred clinical research into the accuracy and precision of diagnostic tests ... the power of prognostic markers and the efficacy and safety of therapeutic, rehabilitative, and preventive regimens' (ibid.).

In relation to this chapter of clinical reasoning and practice epistemology, there are two key issues which need to be addressed pertaining to evidence-based practice: (1) the nature and source of evidence and (2) the notion and the standards for judging best practice. We support the following position in relation to these issues:

- Evidence to support quality practice needs to come from many sources (qualitative as well as quantitative research, experience-based as well as research- and theory-based knowledge). The suitability of the evidence for the type and context of the clinical decision-making or clinical reasoning is what is in question.
- A biopsychosocial model rather than a biomedical model is preferable as the framework for patient-centred clinical practice (Jones et al 2002).
- Best practice is not a simple, absolute, measurable phenomenon. Rather we should seek to provide defensible, optimal, person-centred, context-relevant health care unique to the individual, that is grounded in a range of evidence including propositional and non-propositional (evidence-based) knowledge (Higgs 2000).
- Efficacy (or outcome effectiveness) is one, but not the only, criterion for judging the quality of care. Client preference and choice, the clinician's ability, and quality of life issues during and after the clinical process are also important factors to be addressed (Higgs 2000).
- Reasoning is context-bound. Our understanding of the client's needs and the situation, and our decisions and actions, depend on how well we understand that context. Because of the specificity, uncertainty and complexity of practice there is a need to particularise action (treatments, interventions and collaborative management plans). As professionals dealing with this uncertainty, we rarely apply rigid treatment protocols with blind certainty in unequivocal research-generated knowledge. Actions without thoughtful consideration of the context are habitual rather than professional and do not demonstrate the use of critical thinking or sound knowledge. This is not the intention, nor the ideal, of evidence-based practice.

In order to cope with the complexities and uncertainties of clinical practice (Fig. 11.1) we contend that clinical reasoning needs to be seen as a pivotal

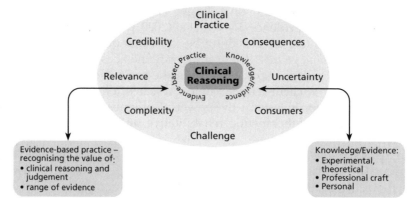

Figure 11.1   Evidence in evidence-based practice and clinical reasoning

point of knowledge management in practice, utilising the principles of evidence-based practice and the findings of research, but also using professional judgement to interpret and make research relevant to the specific patient and the current clinical situation. Practice philosophies and management strategies need to be grounded in a combination of biomedical rationale, broader knowledge of culture and society, clinical experience which has been tested and converted to credible professional knowledge, research knowledge from a variety of research strategies, and clinical evidence or data pertaining to the client's interests. Then we can claim to be adopting credible practice which is not only evidence-based, but also client-centred and context-relevant (Higgs 2000, Jones & Higgs 2000).

Clinical reasoning, judgement artistry and practice knowledge

It is an interesting phenomenon in recent literature that alongside the scientific emphasis of evidence-based practice there is an increasing (re-)discovery and appreciation of professional artistry and practice wisdom. It has been argued that 'professional expertise in the human service professions such as the health professions resides in practice wisdom and practice artistry' (Higgs et al 2001, p. 4). Practice wisdom refers to the possession of practice experience and knowledge, together with the ability to use them critically, intuitively and practically.

Professional artistry can be defined as a creative, advanced way of knowing (and also a way of acting) in practice; it is a deep knowing in practice (Eraut 1985). Such deep knowing represents the epitome of professional judgement and reasoning ability. Professional artistry is exhibited by individuals who possess a blend of artistic and expert qualities built up through extensive and reflective individual knowledge and experience (Beeston &

Higgs 2001). According to Higgs et al (2001, p. 8), professional artistry in practice involves a blend of:

- *practitioner qualities* (e.g. connoisseurship, emotional, physical, existential and spiritual synchronicity and attunement to self, others and what is going on)
- *practice skills* (e.g. expert critical appreciation, ability to disclose or express what has been observed, perceived and done, and metacognitive skills used to balance different domains of professional craft knowledge in the unique care of each client, and to manage the fine interplay between intuition, practical reasoning and rational reasoning and between different kinds of practice knowledge)
- *creative imagination processes* (imagining the outcomes of personalised, unique care interventions and creative strategies to achieve them).

Donald Schön (1983, 1987) was the first of a number of professional educators in recent decades who came to think of professional practice as an artistic endeavour. He called this kind of practice *professional artistry*, proposing that it was valuable to re-examine and develop practice through a careful examination of artistry, which he saw as 'an exercise of intelligence, a kind of knowing, though different in crucial respects from our standard model of professional knowledge' and as 'rigorous in its own terms' (Schön 1987, p. 13). This argument of Schön parallels one of the key notions of clinical reasoning, as a way of knowing (both coming to know or generating knowledge, and using knowledge) in practice, which we present in this chapter.

The epitome of knowing in the creative arts was labelled *connoisseurship* by Eisner (1985), who described this capacity as a way of paying attention. He adopted the accompanying notion of *criticism* as a way of disclosing or expressing what had been seen and considered, arguing that both these elements are essential to artists if they are to contribute to their art in ways that have impact and produce change. Similarly, Fish (1998) contended that the development of professional artistry requires attention to the dimensions of practice which are often invisible: the values, beliefs, attitudes, assumptions, expectations, feelings and knowledge which lie below the surface and behind the actions of practitioners; this is also reflected in their personal knowledge. This argument reflects that of Benner et al (1996), who recognised the place of Aristotelian practical reasoning in expert clinical judgement. The value of professional artistry in relation to practice epistemology is that it requires practitioners to mediate propositional, professional craft and personal knowledge in the messy world of practice, to realise practical principles and use the whole self therapeutically (Benner et al 1996). Professional artistry can be said to be 'the meaningful expression of a uniquely individual view within a shared tradition' (Beeston & Higgs 2001, p. 114). Although such practice may be expressed as something uniquely individual, it is not individualistic; it requires a context characterised by continuing development and sharing of all forms of knowledge within a community of practice.

CLINICAL REASONING AS A VEHICLE FOR THE DEVELOPMENT OF THE KNOWLEDGE BASE OF THE PROFESSION AND THE PRACTITIONER

Clinical reasoning is inherently a vehicle for acquisition and development of knowledge as well as decision-making. Both the implementation of sound clinical reasoning and the generation of knowledge through reasoning involve practitioners in:

- continually expanding and refining their knowledge bases
- translating their practice 'knowings' into articulable knowledge
- learning in action and testing their knowledge during reasoning
- developing a deep understanding of the procedural knowledge and processes underlying clinical reasoning and seeking to develop knowledge and reasoning through critical appraisal and testing of emerging reasoning strategies
- constantly challenging and developing the various interpersonal and clinical skills (e.g. physical examination procedures) that provide input to or facilitate clinical reasoning in action.

Professionals are exhorted and taught to engage in lifelong learning, to enhance continually (and update) their knowledge content and their competence. During clinical reasoning, clinicians can become aware of the deficiencies of their knowledge bases by recognising that some knowledge areas or advances seem unfamiliar and realising that in some tasks their knowledge seems inadequate, inaccurate or insufficient. In addition to ongoing review of knowledge content, clinical reasoning prompts clinicians to assess the utility, relevance and adequacy of their knowledge structure. Because of the need for sound decision-making with the aim of providing best practice for the individual client, knowledge testing is essential. In part this occurs as an ongoing responsibility so that learning can inform future practice. Testing of knowledge in a variety of contexts clarifies the situations in which particular actions are appropriate or inappropriate. Without this critical analysis there is a danger of actions becoming routinised and performed uncritically (Baskett et al 1992).

Within practice, critical appraisal occurs at the metacognitive level. Metacognition, or reflective self-awareness, allows clinicians to monitor the quality of information obtained, evaluate the limitations in their knowledge and thinking and detect unexpected findings (e.g. clinical data which do not fit the emerging clinical pattern, or clinical pictures which challenge long-held certainties). Such dissonance raises questions for individual clinicians about the soundness, adequacy, scope and depth of their knowledge bases, and also raises questions for research or practice exploration.

CONCLUSION

Credible and accountable clinical decisions rely on a number of forms of knowledge and evidence. This evidence includes professional craft knowledge and research knowledge derived from across the range of research methods, including experimental, interpretive and action research. Credible evidence of many forms is needed to serve the complementary tasks of performing clinical reasoning and engaging in evidence-based practice within the complex, uncertain world of professional practice. In this chapter we have examined clinical reasoning (including the use of professional judgement and practice knowledge in clinical decision-making) and its relationship with practice knowledge and practice epistemology. In essence, clinical reasoning is a means of allowing knowledge and evidence to inform and be tested and generated through practice.

REFERENCES

Alexander, P. A. & Judy, J. E. (1988). The interaction of domain-specific and strategic knowledge in academic performance. *Review of Educational Research*, **58**, 375–404.
Arocha, J. F., Patel, V. L. & Patel, Y. C. (1993). Hypothesis generation and the coordination of theory and evidence in novice diagnostic reasoning. *Medical Decision-Making*, **13**, 198–211.
Barnitt, R. (1998). Ethical dilemmas in occupational therapy and physical therapy: a survey of practitioners in the UK National Health Services. *Journal of Medical Ethics*, **24**, 193–9.
Baskett, H. K. M., Marsick, V. J. & Cervero, R. M. (1992). Putting theory to practice and practice to theory. In *Professions' Ways of Knowing: New Findings on How to Improve Professional Education* (H. K. M. Baskett & V. J. Marsick, eds) pp. 109–18. San Francisco: Jossey-Bass.
Basseches, M. (1984). *Dialectical Thinking and Adult Development*. Norwood, NJ: Ablex.
Beeston, S. & Higgs, J. (2001). Professional practice: artistry and connoisseurship. In *Practice Knowledge and Expertise in the Health Professions* (J. Higgs & A. Titchen, eds) pp. 108–17. Oxford: Butterworth-Heinemann.
Benner, P. (1984). *From Novice to Expert: Excellence and Power in Clinical Nursing Practice*. London: Addison-Wesley.
Benner, P. (1991). The role of experience, narrative, and community in skilled ethical comportment. *Advances in Nursing Science*, **14**, 1–21.
Benner, P. & Tanner, C. (1987). Clinical judgement: how expert nurses use intuition. *American Journal of Nursing*, **87**, 23–31.
Benner, P., Tanner, C. & Chesla, C. (1996). *Expertise in Nursing Practice: Caring, Clinical Judgement and Ethics*. New York: Springer.
Boshuizen, H. P. A. & Schmidt, H. G. (2000). The development of clinical reasoning expertise. In *Clinical Reasoning in the Health Professions*, 2nd edn (J. Higgs & M. Jones, eds) pp. 15–22. Oxford: Butterworth-Heinemann.
Burke, J. P. & DePoy, E. (1991). An emerging view of mastery, excellence, and leadership in occupational therapy practice. *American Journal of Occupational Therapy*, **45**(11), 1027–32.
Dreyfus, H. L. & Dreyfus, S. E. (1986). *Mind Over Machine*. New York: The Free Press.
Edwards, I. (2001). *Clinical Reasoning in Three Different Fields of Physiotherapy: A Qualitative Case Study*. Unpublished PhD thesis. Adelaide: University of South Australia.
Eisner, E. (1985). *The Art of Educational Evaluation: A Personal View*. London: Falmer Press.

Elstein, A. S., Shulman, L. S. & Sprafka, S. A. (1978). *Medical Problem-Solving: An Analysis of Clinical Reasoning*. Cambridge, MA: Harvard University Press.

Elstein, A. S., Shulman, L. & Sprafka, S. (1990). Medical problem-solving: a ten year retrospective. *Evaluation and the Health Professions*, **13**(1), 5–36.

Eraut, M. (1985). Knowledge creation and knowledge use in professional contexts. *Studies in Higher Education*, **10**(2), 117–33.

Eraut, M. (1994). *Developing Professional Knowledge and Competence*. London: Falmer Press.

Fish, D. (1998). *Appreciating Practice in the Caring Professions: Refocusing Professional Development and Practitioner Research*. Oxford: Butterworth-Heinemann.

Fleming, M. H. (1991). The therapist with the three track mind. *American Journal of Occupational Therapy*, **45**, 1007–14.

Gastmans, C., Dierckx de Casterle, B. & Schotsmans, P. (1998). Nursing considered as moral practice: a philosophical–ethical interpretation of nursing. *Kennedy Institute of Ethics Journal*, **8**, 43–69.

Glaser, R. & Chi, M. T. H. (1988). Overview. In *The Nature of Expertise* (M. T. H. Chi, R. Glaser & M. J. Farr, eds) pp. xvi–xxviii. Hillsdale, NJ: Lawrence Erlbaum Associates.

Gordon, M., Murphy, C. P., Candee, D. & Hiltunen, E. (1994). Clinical judgement: an integrated model. *Advances in Nursing Science*, **16**, 55–70.

Grant, J. & Marsden, P. (1987). The structure of memorized knowledge in students and clinicians: an explanation for diagnostic expertise. *Medical Education*, **21**, 92–8.

Hagedorn, R. (1996). Clinical decision-making in familiar cases: a model of the process and implications for practice. *British Journal of Occupational Therapy*, **59**, 217–22.

Higgs, J. (2000). Evidence-based practice: interpreting, producing and justifying evidence. In *Congress Proceedings, The Sixth International Physiotherapy Congress*, pp. 61–63. Canberra: Australian Physiotherapy Association.

Higgs, J. & Jones, M. (2000). Clinical reasoning in the health professions. In *Clinical Reasoning in the Health Professions*, 2nd edn (J. Higgs & M. Jones, eds) pp. 3–14. Oxford: Butterworth-Heinemann.

Higgs, J., Titchen, A. & Neville, V. (2001). Professional practice and knowledge. In *Practice Knowledge and Expertise in the Health Professions* (J. Higgs & A. Titchen, eds) pp. 3–9. Oxford: Butterworth-Heinemann.

Jensen, G. M., Shepard, K. F., Gwyer, J. & Hack, L. M. (1992). Attribute dimensions that distinguish master and novice physical therapy clinicians in orthopedic settings. *Physical Therapy*, **72**(10), 711–22.

Jensen, G. M., Gwyer, J., Hack, L. M. & Shepard, K. F. (1999). *Expertise in Physical Therapy Practice*. Boston: Butterworth-Heinemann.

Jones, J. A. (1988). Clinical reasoning in nursing. *Journal of Advanced Nursing*, **13**, 185–92.

Jones, M. & Higgs, J. (2000). Will evidence-based practice take the reasoning out of practice? In *Clinical Reasoning in the Health Professions*, 2nd edn (J. Higgs & M. Jones, eds) pp. 307–15. Oxford: Butterworth-Heinemann.

Jones, M. A., Jensen, G. & Edwards, I. (2000). Clinical reasoning in physiotherapy. In *Clinical Reasoning in the Health Professions*, 2nd edn (J. Higgs & M. A. Jones, eds) pp. 117–27. Oxford: Butterworth-Heinemann.

Jones, M., Edwards, I. & Gifford, L. (2002). Conceptual models for implementing biopsychosocial theory in clinical practice. *Manual Therapy*, **7**(1), 2–9.

Lorig, K. R., Sobel, D. S., Stewart, A. L. et al (1999). Evidence suggesting that a chronic disease self-management program can improve health status while reducing utilization and costs: a randomised trial. *Medical Care*, **37**, 5–14.

Mattingly, C. (1991). The narrative nature of clinical reasoning. *American Journal of Occupational Therapy*, **45**, 998–1005.

Mattingly, C. & Hayes Fleming, M. (1994). *Clinical Reasoning: Forms of Inquiry in a Therapeutic Practice*. Philadelphia: F. A. Davis.

Mezirow, J. (1991). *Transformative Dimensions of Adult Learning*. San Francisco: Jossey-Bass.

Nicholas, B. & Gillett, G. (1997). Doctors' stories, patients' stories: a narrative approach to teaching medical ethics. *Journal of Medical Ethics*, **23**, 295–9.

Nicholls, D. (2000). Breathlessness: a qualitative model of meaning. *Physiotherapy*, **86**(1), 23–7.

Nickerson, R. S., Perkins, D. N. & Smith, E. E. (1985). *The Teaching of Thinking*. Hillsdale, NJ: Lawrence Erlbaum Associates.

O'Loughlin, A. (1999). On living with chronic pain. In *Nursing and the Experience of Illness: Phenomenology in Practice* (I. Madjar & J. A. Walton, eds) pp. 123–44. Australia: Allen & Unwin.

Patel, V. L. & Groen, G. J. (1986). Knowledge based solution strategies in medical reasoning. *Cognitive Science*, **10**, 91–116.

Paterson, M. & Higgs, J. (2001). *Professional Practice Judgement Artistry.* Occasional paper 3. Sydney: Centre for Professional Education Advancement, University of Sydney.

Payton, O. D. (1985). Clinical reasoning process in physical therapy. *Physical Therapy*, **65**, 924–8.

Radovich, S. (2001). Innovations in school-based intervention: an overview of a school-based model of service delivery and clinical education. *Australian Communication Quarterly*, **31**, 23–5.

Rew, L. & Barrow, E. (1987). Intuition: a neglected hallmark of nursing knowledge. *Advances in Nursing Science*, **10**(1), 49–62.

Rogers, J. C. & Masagatani, G. (1982). Clinical reasoning of occupational therapists during the initial assessment of physically disabled patients. *Occupational Therapy Journal of Research*, **2**, 195–219.

Sackett, D. L., Straus, S. E., Richardson, W. S., Rosenberg, W. & Haynes, R. B. (2000). *Evidence-Based Medicine: How to Practice and Teach EBM*, 2nd edn. London: Churchill Livingstone.

Schell, B. A. & Cervero, R. M. (1993). Clinical reasoning in occupational therapy: an integrative review. *American Journal of Occupational Therapy*, **47**, 605–10.

Schmidt, H. G. & Boshuizen, H. P. A. (1993). On acquiring expertise in medicine. *Educational Psychology Review*, **5**, 205–21.

Schmidt, H. G., Boshuizen, H. P. A. & Norman, G. R. (1992). Reflections on the nature of expertise in medicine. In *Deep Models for Medical Knowledge Engineering* (E. Keravnou, ed.) pp. 231–48. Amsterdam: Elsevier.

Schön, D. A. (1983). *The Reflective Practitioner: How Professionals Think in Action.* London: Temple Smith.

Schön, D. A. (1987). *Educating the Reflective Practitioner.* San Francisco: Jossey-Bass.

Sim, J. (1998). Respect for autonomy: issues in neurological rehabilitation. *Clinical Rehabilitation*, **12**, 3–10.

Stewart, M. & Brown, J. B. (2001). Patient-centredness in medicine. In *Evidence-Based Patient Choice* (A. Edwards & G. Elwyn, eds) pp. 97–117. Oxford: Oxford University Press.

Titchen, A. (2000). *Professional Craft Knowledge in Patient-Centred Nursing and the Facilitation of its Development.* University of Oxford DPhil thesis. Oxford: Ashdale Press.

White, K. (2001). Professional craft knowledge and ethical decision-making. In *Practice Knowledge and Expertise in the Health Professions* (J. Higgs & A. Titchen, eds) pp. 142–8. Oxford: Butterworth-Heinemann.

White, M. & Epston, D. (1990). *Narrative Means to Therapeutic Ends.* New York: W. W. Norton.

12

Practice epistemology: implications for education, practice and research

Barbara Richardson, Madeleine Abrandt Dahlgren and Joy Higgs

INTRODUCTION

In this chapter we take a summary view of the wide range of dimensions of epistemology revealed through the chapters in this book, conceptualising professional practice as it would look within a full understanding of the knowledge that underpins it. In doing so we identify a number of implications for education, practice and research. From these we then examine ways in which our practice can be further explained and characterised to maximise its potential and its contribution to health. We conclude with a forward look at some social trends and structures that may influence the ongoing evolution of professional practice. We aim to present the reader with ideas, possibilities and challenges to answer the anticipated questions, 'Where to from here?' and 'What does this mean for my practice/teaching/research?'

WHAT DO WE KNOW ABOUT THE KNOWLEDGE NEEDED FOR HEALTH CARE?

Although the different chapters deal with somewhat different aspects of practice knowledge, one feature that comes through clearly in all chapters is the ontological perspective of health care. The ontological perspective concerns our view of the nature of the world, or of a phenomenon in the world like health care. The ontological perspective put forward in this book portrays health care as an *idiographic* field of knowledge of many dimensions, which does not comply fully with the *nomothetic* ideals of the natural sciences. Nagel (1961) described the distinction between '[the nomothetic] which seeks to establish abstract general laws for indefinitely repeatable events and processes; and the ideographic, which aims to understand the unique and nonrecurrent' (p. 547). Nagel suggested that Aristotle is the source of this distinction, but attributed the terms to the German philosopher Wilhelm Windelband (1915).

Why then is it important to talk about ontological perspectives in a book on practice epistemology? We argue that it is important to be aware that how you view the world is dependent on how you conceptualise the possibilities for achieving knowledge about it: that is, the relation between ontological and epistemological questions and issues. In that sense, this book replicates the critique, by Schön and others, that rejects the view of technical rationality as the sole knowledge base for health care professionals. The chapters of this book collectively demonstrate that the knowledge for professional practice is created from reflection on those perspectives of practice that practitioners believe are central to their daily work. Our authors suggest that the sense of 'knowing' about practice is developed, refined and defined in the communities of practice in which practitioners work, in which they share a common understanding of the activities considered to be central to practice, a common understanding of what counts as knowledge and how it should be critically appraised and appreciated. An epistemology of practice thus incorporates all these sources of knowledge, and its development is interdependent with development of practice. We cannot fully recognise an inclusive epistemology of practice without first appreciating all the sources of knowing that we encounter in daily practice, and we cannot appreciate the full knowledge base from which we work until we seriously consider the range of sources of knowledge which are involved in creating practice knowledge.

Central to our argument of the value of articulating and using practice epistemology, as a way of doing and developing practice, is the understanding that knowledge of professional practice is generated by practitioners themselves in interaction with others in practical social activities. Within the social context of health care, interactions with others include direct interaction with people and indirect interaction with systems of work, organisations, imposed regulations for ethical behaviour, financial constraints and policies relating to working strictly within interpreted frameworks of evidence-based medicine. All these influences can have an impact on practice decision-making and thus have implications for the outcomes of our interventions. The ways in which practitioners visualise the boundaries of professional knowledge are reflected in the way they reason clinically, make decisions, keep records and carry out their assessments and evaluations. Together these actions demonstrate to the practitioners and to others in the health care team their understanding of the extent of the professional knowledge on which they base their practice.

We believe the full contribution of this book is that it has advanced this stated position on professional knowledge. We have articulated several dimensions of knowledge that have implications when brought into the reflections of practitioners themselves. Key claims in this book are that increased awareness of different sources of knowledge, a sensitivity for the idiosyncratic and reflective collaboration with peers are hallmarks for building a knowledge base that is explicit and that can reveal dimensions of knowledge which already function tacitly as valid. Many of the chapters contain elegant arguments for attention to a number of such perspectives. The production of professional knowledge is thus seen as something pertaining to the activities of every professional practitioner, not something that is executed exclusively by scientists. The challenge lies in integrating this understanding of professional knowledge into daily professional practice and in how practitioners view their role in contributing to the knowledge of their profession.

WHAT WOULD PRACTICE LOOK LIKE THAT IS CARRIED OUT BY PROFESSIONALS WHO KNOW ABOUT KNOWING?

In optimal professional practice, it is natural for professionals to enter into dialogue, with both their peers and their students, about their knowledge of what they are doing or planning to do, and to reason with them about why they judge their knowledge use to be valid in a specific case. As discussed in this book, the need for documenting and writing about one's observations is of course of paramount importance, but equally important is the need to articulate knowledge orally. It is through verbalising their knowledge that practitioners become aware of the strengths and weaknesses of their reasoning and of the claims they make. We aim in this book to replace a position of giving primacy to theory with a recognition of the inherent primacy of practice, and we hope also to challenge traditional views that the written word is comprehensively more important and valid than the spoken word when it comes to claims of knowledge. In this regard evidence-based medicine becomes paradoxical. It developed with the aims of reinforcing practitioners' work and enhancing the quality of health care with the best available knowledge to inform their practices. However, in many cases it is likely that it has had the opposite effect, and has instead silenced practitioners and weakened professionals' confidence in discussing the legitimate contribution of their clinical skills and practice knowledge to their practice.

Practitioners' critical conversations with peers in their own and other professions

The importance of articulating practice knowledge verbally is strongly emphasised. It is the first step towards colleagues being able to scrutinise critically the rationale for the choices and decisions practitioners make in the clinical encounter. Talking about clinical reasoning will help consolidate and legitimise the nature and extent of the knowledge generated and applied in practice. If practitioners engage in critical conversations of this type with peers within and across health care teams and with the users of health care, the patients, they can begin to tease out the clinical, ethical and moral reasoning that they have undertaken. Consciously or unconsciously such sequences of reasoning, of cognitive action, underpin every professional action. The complexity of the reasoning, the way practitioners think, forms the basis of their individual expertise and that which distinguishes them from others in their profession and from other professionals in the health care team. Each practitioner works in this way, with different perspectives and experiences that together can contribute to and deepen the pool of practice knowledge.

The consequences of practice actions may not always be uppermost in the minds of practitioners, either during interactions with individual patients or during broader activities that can influence society at large. Yet such consequences do arise. For example, the decision to focus on cure or rehabilitation rather than actively to promote health with one patient or one group of patients may reinforce an understanding that this particular profession is not involved with health promotion. This perception may in turn lead to some professions not being considered or invited to participate as stakeholders in health developments in the local or national arena. Engaging in critical conversations with peers, students and others can provide a way to determine which care processes are thought to be effective and which need research to investigate their effectiveness. Discussion within individual professional groups can examine the relevance, safety and efficacy of techniques and approaches that are unique to or prominent within a particular profession. Multidisciplinary groups can examine the efficacy of combined approaches for specific patient groups within the confines of allocated resources and facilities. This is the starting point from which further epistemological perspectives can arise through practice development and from which education and research can take direction for future initiatives.

Mixing together different types of knowledge to draw on a range of sources of information

Optimal professional practice can occur when practitioners take all kinds of sources of knowledge into account in the clinical situation and make use of them wisely for their specific goals. We do not reject the idea that knowledge can be produced according to the hypothetico-deductive model, we simply argue that practitioners need to become aware that this is only one perspective of what counts as knowledge. In practice settings, much of the work of a successful encounter rests on how practitioners actually utilise the knowledge produced through hypothetico-deductive processes. This includes how they take the extant knowledge of books and research papers and use it in the different modes of application they select, taking into account the physical, social, ethical and moral factors of the specific health care situation. In pointing out alternative ways of producing and appreciating knowledge we argue that they are equally valid and essential to practice effectiveness. Time for reflection on practice, time for metacognition to monitor thinking in practice, lies at the heart of recognising the validity of new experiential knowledge and continuing to reappraise the validity of older accepted and given knowledge. This profound and demanding activity is part of establishing the quality, currency and justification of treatments and approaches used in health care in relation to contemporary needs. General observation of policies aimed to increase patients' involvement in their health care, of moves to increase physical activity in societies, and of other strategies to increase community participation in healthy lifestyles calls into question many of the passive treatments and interventions in health care that are professionally labour-intensive, of high cost, and tending to create patient dependency.

Giving help to build research studies which can effectively examine practice

This book indicates that optimal practice occurs when practitioners acknowledge their responsibilities in highlighting the need for research into specific areas of practice and where possible become engaged in research that can explore critical issues of their practice. While academics can provide the structured background of carrying out research studies which are valid, reliable and ethically conducted, practitioners can best explain the likely key interacting features. Practitioners can provide a working understanding of difficulties in terminology between lay people and professionals, and can unravel and articulate their praxis (that is, the mental and physical processes they engage in when carrying out their practice). Only a full explication of practice, often developed through processes of qualitative research or action research, can provide those who will carry out the research with sufficient detail to design high-quality research studies that can make a definitive contribution to human knowledge.

Practitioners' engagement in the continuum of education of themselves and others

A notion of a dynamic, fluid process of knowledge creation at the centre of everyday practice need not change the way practitioners put their practice into action, but it will encourage them to broaden their thinking and to focus on exactly what they are doing. If we accept it as axiomatic that practice is a key avenue for generating knowledge or basic truth, we establish a fresh view of the activities of practice and how they can inform research and education. In many ways practice can be regarded as part of the continuum of education. Through practice, new things can be learned each day in relation to patients, the professional role, colleagues, the community and the health care system. The ways in which practitioners recognise such information and how it is dealt with as part of the learning process are among the most crucial aspects of fieldwork experience for students and of early professional work of novice staff. Experience of the reality of professional practice cannot be gained from the classroom. Retrospective reflection by students on clinical reasoning processes shown in videos or when they are working with colleagues in classroom contexts, although of enormous importance to their learning process, can never replace the immediacy, complexity and humanity of events in the clinical setting which lead to practice outcomes. Discussion and explication of how these are managed and incorporated in day-to-day work are of immense value to students and junior professionals to assist in the development of their reasoning processes.

Optimal organisation of practice which acknowledges the validity of all the sources of professional knowledge will ensure that workloads and work diaries show time for self-reflection on personal development; time to draw together with peers to reflect on all the sources of information used in interactions with a patient, a patient group, or in working with a practice intervention; time for collaboration and reflection with others in the health care team on treatment practices; time for collaboration with colleagues in research; and time for education and supervision of other members of the professional group and in health care generally. Purposeful management of time as a valuable health care resource is fundamental to ensure that practitioners are able to contribute fully to the further development and use of professional knowledge. Department managers have an important role in establishing a culture of a community of practice in which trees do not obscure the view of the wood. Practice communities need to maintain a firm focus on the interaction of the profession with the social world of which they form a part, as well as on providing the day-to-day delivery of health care. The modes of knowledge generation and application carried out in practice settings are replicated in the wider processes of interaction which incorporate the views and expectations of other stakeholders in health care, including service purchasers and the public, to ensure that each relevant profession is at the leading edge in health and social care development. In this respect reducing a waiting list may seem less important than understanding why it has arisen in the first place.

Optimal organisation of practice is shown in the level of clinical governance of health care resources. This includes the management of resources, in collaboration with other health professionals, in systems of access to service and in timely and appropriate appointments made available to patients. Optimal organisation of practice is further demonstrated when practitioners engage in activities in which they acknowledge themselves as members of the wider community of their profession's practice and recognise the interdependence of research, practice and education activities in the generation and application of professional knowledge. Research activities may include participating in research planning groups to refine research questions, developing protocols for data collection and collecting data. Research can also involve departmental policies of recording patient information in ways that provide full and accurate baseline measurements and information, and discharge assessments that evaluate interventions and patient responses, that can later be retrieved as research data. Educational activities can include supervision of undergraduate or postgraduate students in collaboration with academic institutes as well as supervision of staff development through appraisal and mentoring systems. Whether they are explicit or covert, many opportunities can be provided which encourage enthusiasm for enquiry, discussion and debate to flourish at all levels of practice.

In summary, optimal practice is based on practitioners' understanding of the key role practice plays in the generation and development of their professional knowledge and of the resulting equal attention they pay to their treatment and to reflection and collaboration with others. If this view of practice was commonly adopted, health professionals could examine more closely how the practice of each profession could be further explained, described or characterised, and they could consider the implications for the development and expansion of professional knowledge to ensure best practice of health care.

WHAT MORE CAN BE DONE TO EXPLAIN AND CHARACTERISE PRACTICE KNOWLEDGE?

If we consider what we agree to be the nature of professional knowledge, the ways in which we acquire it and the ways in which we use it, it becomes clear how it can be further explained and characterised by the concept of a continuum of practice, education and research. It also becomes clear that there is a constant need for practitioners to replenish the stock of knowledge on which practice is based, so that it reflects the contemporary needs of health care and can ensure a quality and cost-effective service to all clients.

Professional practice can be better understood and described in practice settings

As a phenomenon that continually develops through practice by building on appraisal of the knowledge used in practice, professional knowledge can be regarded as a process as well as a product. Knowing in professional practice is a process that is fed, energised and driven by individuals in their work, but its momentum can be maintained only through making it explicit: through talking about it and reflecting on it with others in professional debate. In that way some ideas are discarded and others reinforced through the normal processes of social interaction and peer review. We all have a responsibility to share our thoughts and the reasons for our actions in practice. Through detailing practice activities and analysing them together, new knowledge can be identified and old knowledge can be developed or abandoned as no longer relevant. An example of the latter is the knowledge related to the management of people who are handicapped. This area of knowledge has been influenced by the recent major recategorisation of disability and functioning by the World Health Organization (WHO) (2001), that has moved the focus away from the concept of handicap to the knowledge needed by professionals to enable people to function optimally in their environments. By reflecting on such changes in knowing and knowledge, practitioners are able to consider more fully how their practice contributes to contemporary health needs, and the research and educational activities that are needed to support it.

Reforming practice requires a transformation of people's understanding of the basic assumptions of their practice and practice research (Desforges 2001). It requires us to take a sceptical view of actions in practice and to maintain an open mind as to their worth and validity in the context of changing settings and health care demands. An ability to disengage from the immediate professional action and to take a longer view of professional behaviour in the broadening fields of health care is one of the cornerstones of professional thinking, distinguishing it from the technical thinking that follows procedures unquestioningly. Further illumination of these views can lead to a more precise characterisation of practice. Views on practice discussed with critical friends, on an individual level or in professional groups gain a wider appraisal and can be placed within the context of new research evidence, new health care policies and the emergence of new patient groups. Such changes can help to motivate and enable practitioners to keep abreast of learning that can maximise their clinical effectiveness. With regard to implementing evidence-based practice, there is a role for practitioners in providing protected time for support that can help develop the level of 'research receptivity' in practitioners (Bond 2002, p. 237) and their ability to interpret research findings and apply them to their practice. Such people can facilitate and encourage the professional debate that helps to articulate how research findings are integrated with experiential practice knowledge. In addition to regular 'journal clubs' to promote peer review of recent published papers, practitioners and managers can encourage a culture of continual critical appraisal of research and practice, to answer questions posed by practitioners and to help increase their confidence in their research self-efficacy (Bond 2002).

Collaborative work in health care has numerous advantages. It can optimise patient referral patterns so that the effect of long waiting lists in terms of negative outcomes of practice can be minimised. Recording patient information can provide useful data for clinical or cost-effectiveness studies. Enhanced multidisciplinary working interactions facilitate and clarify the goals of client-focused care which in turn can help to sharpen knowledge used and needed in practice (including knowledge supporting cultural competence and the depth of the client's knowledge). Practitioners are said to require flexibility as a core capability (Broadbent et al 1977, p. 7).

Health care policies can serve to spearhead critical debate on professional knowledge and its origins. Evidence-based practice is an example of this process. It has influenced some people (Jones & Higgs 2000, Johnstone & Lacey 2002) to challenge research-limited definitions of evidence and to identify the need for experience-generated knowledge to be included in definitions for evidence for best practice. Importantly, such knowledge/evidence is not just a gap-filler in areas where research knowledge fails to supply answers for clinical decision-making. Professional craft knowledge provides core evidence and direction to support and guide the humanity, variability and essential quality of best professional practice.

Sophisticated communication systems are making variations in practice and intervention outcome more visible in many professions, and it is important to show how the professional task is one that requires the exercise of discretion or initiative on behalf of another in a situation of complexity (Eve & Hodgkin 1997, p. 71) and to reflect on agreed good practice. Many of the new regulatory systems are creating changes in clinical freedom. In particular, the effects of traditionally hidden financial pressures are becoming more visible, and careful justification of practice is needed to ensure the ratification of professional decision-making as clinically and cost-effective. Such policies of accountability and justification can benefit from analysis of the components of professional knowledge and evaluation of their contribution.

What can be done further to describe and explain practice through education?

Habits of reflection and open debate on all practice issues are at the foundation of practice and of learning through practice. Professional education is a lifelong process of construction of knowledge, in which the benefits of sharing views at each stage are recognised. Orientation of student practitioners to this line of thinking is incumbent on the education programmes and the practitioners and supervisors involved in education. A basic understanding of the shared process that leads to the development, application and utilisation of practice knowledge in each health care problem is fundamental. Educational or curriculum goals which recognise the important influences of socialisation in the explicit and informal curriculum are important (Richardson et al 2002) to ensure links between the classroom and practice.

Socialisation, the explicit and covert ways in which new members of a profession learn to be like other professionals and to be accepted members of the profession, provides an avenue that can drive the continual search for professional knowledge for each profession. Clearly the prime context for this is the practice setting. Practitioners, supervisors and managers bear an awesome responsibility for encouraging workplace cultures that are conducive to promoting an enquiring and critical nature in future practitioners, and for supporting those who have returned to formal education in widening their expertise and understanding of their profession. This is not always an easy task, and it is one that can be seriously curtailed by individual practitioners feeling threatened rather than pleased about taking a wide view of the responsibility to contribute to practice development. A modern prerequisite of practice is a disposition to learning cooperatively (Desforges 2001, p. 33). This capacity can be enhanced by computer and media literacy, which fosters such processes. Using these skills, practitioners can explore patient-visited websites that can be added to a critical overview of professional knowledge, increasing the understanding of how knowledge is disseminated to lay and professional groups. Adaptability and creativity in clinical judgements, showing practitioners' wisdom in appreciation of the number of sources of knowledge available, are vital to effective communication with patients and peers.

Practitioners' understanding of the processes of building new knowledge can help students of all levels to capitalise on the interactions between formal teaching and practice experiences (Bereiter & Scardamalia 1996, cited in Desforges 2001). The challenge of teaching processes which deal with anomalous information, that is, information which is unexpected and which can lead to a disequilibrium of confidence (Desforges 2001, p. 9), is a key issue in building new knowledge for professionals, clinical supervisors and tutors. The very notion of professional knowledge as an individually

and socially constructed phenomenon should give practitioners an awareness of involvement with education on many fronts: with patients, with
students, with colleagues of all levels of seniority and experience, and with
others in the health care team. There will be something to learn from each of
these educational interactions, which can then be modified or built upon in
other experiences. Reflecting the importance of communication in health
care and in knowledge development, such interactions offer a rich field
from which to identify topics for research, as well as personal quests of
meaning-making from practice.

A move by the National Health Service (UK), one of the greatest health care
employers in Europe, away from organisational hierarchies of management
to management webs of action in focused care groups (Eve & Hodgkin 1997)
heralds a redesign of systems of care in which professional practice opportunities will be dependent upon who is involved in these microsystems of care
and who are the key players. Organisational models of web management are
considered to facilitate a broadening of knowledge and its applicability to
specific tasks. Involvement in such systems to ensure that the profession's
voice is heard is important, but keeping a profession-specific focus within a
health care team can be difficult. Such contexts require integration of ideas
together with the capacity to present reasoned arguments for profession-
specific practices (Centre for the Advancement of Interprofessional Education 2002, p. 34). Reflective and critical conversations in within-profession
groups, away from the health care team, are essential for the development of
that profession's practice, and also as a means of reviewing decision-making
processes that may have become too dogmatic to incorporate new practice.
It is important to reflect on the processes of health care as well as its outcome. Development of a role for critical companions and clinical mentors
(Tompson & Ryan 1996, Titchen 2000) will be of great assistance in responding to the call for reflection that can link to creating and legitimising an epistemology of practice (Schön 1995).

Professional knowledge development in multidisciplinary teams relies
on an agreed need for continuous quality improvement to find better ways
of meeting the needs of patients or clients (Wilcock 1998a). Increasingly, a
systems view of processes of care, in which the perspectives of all team
members can be heard and valued, enables the tacit knowledge and expertise of each team member to be acknowledged in the overall management of
the client. This systems approach, in which each person is seen to contribute to overall team performance, is particularly evident in the area of
patient safety. Here, microsystems of work are identified which are considered to be safe systems within which patient safety risks can more easily
be assessed (Barach & Moss 2001). Team members are encouraged not only
to strive to a shared understanding of how each directly or indirectly affects
the delivery of care to patients, but also to have an overview of the work-
ings of the total system of health care. These dual understandings can help

health professionals to appreciate how health care can affect the patho-logical progress of patient problems along with the quality of their lives. It has been suggested that most human system problems lie in processes rather than people (Wilcock 1998a). Exploring together how processes of care delivery currently work can facilitate improvements in effectiveness and efficiency of care (Wilcock 1998b). Such activities can also provide an opportunity for articulation of the details of practice. All practitioners must act as advocates for their own health care focus. Systems of access, for example, are often based on a linear view of patients being managed through a system which primarily proceeds from general practitioner to consultants and back again, with the authority and decision-making resid-ing in those two roles. Strong core management support is needed to achieve integration of primary, secondary and community care, both in aligning financial and quality incentives and in eliminating inappropriate organisational barriers. However, each practitioner should be able to con-tribute to discussion of professional contributions, raise awareness and drive improvements forward.

What can be done further to describe and explain practice through research?

The move towards evidence-based practice provides an impetus for all prac-titioners to examine their practice. This can become a demoralising process when it is realised that so little professional practice has been researched and that existing research is often considered to be of such poor quality that little evidence can be gleaned from it for generalisation. A key to coping with this dilemma is an ability to take a clear, cool look at all the aspects of practice that appear in the contributions of different research approaches. It is import-ant to differentiate clearly approaches when critiquing research and also when generating questions of practice that research can help to examine. The more clearly the nature of practice activities and their underlying knowledge can be described to highlight the areas needing research, the more rigorous the research design and approach will be. It is crucial, then, for practitioners to act as ambassadors for the range of knowledge types incorporated in their practice. Clinical reasoning and reflection on practice shared in critical conversations with others form a platform from which practitioners can expound the ontological perspective within which they work and the range of knowledge required to support it. To gain acceptance of this perspective of practice and its contribution to health care, we need to provide convincing arguments to colleagues who are yet to appreciate the value and legitimacy of practice and the range of research activities that can support it. The implications of the challenge of this expanded awareness cannot be overestimated, since for many it will require fundamental changes in the knowledge assumptions on which they currently base their practice.

Knowledge of how to promulgate an appreciation of the 'intersubjectivity' of explanations of health care processes is sorely needed and could be, although it has not yet been, encompassed in the development of cultural theories of education (Desforges 2001, p. 25). Such theories could provide a basis for discussion further to expand and categorise knowledge for health care. The involvement in research of practitioners, patients and carers is critical to knowledge development in practice. It is particularly important for patients to understand the need for them to participate in long-term follow-up studies, and to feel able to raise research questions themselves.

The scope for further development of practice and professional knowledge is endless; it is as broad as the changes in the societies of which health care services are a part. The need for a knowledge of knowledge for practice will be continually with us, and alerts us to consider what may help or hinder its development.

WHAT ARE SOME OF THE SOCIAL TRENDS AND STRUCTURES OF PRACTICE THAT MAY INFLUENCE FURTHER EVOLUTION OF PROFESSIONAL KNOWLEDGE DEVELOPMENT?

A number of changes emerging in society have implications for practice epistemology, highlighting the need for continued development of professional knowledge. These changes range from new answers to the perpetual question about what professions actually contribute to the health of a society, to the changes in outlook and lifestyles involving increasing use of cyberspace and electronic communication.

Is the professional contribution to health obvious?

If there is a need for motivation to think about knowing about knowledge for practice, it is timely to consider the ongoing debate about whether professions show the capability of solving individual health problems. It is suggested that if in industrial societies we are successfully solving health problems, there must be higher levels of disease in traditional preindustrial peoples, who should suffer from a greater number of unresolved diseases (Goldsmith 1999). However, this is not the case. Many live long lives free from disease, particularly cancer. The increasing incidence of cancer suggests it to be primarily induced by the conditions and methods of modern living (Hoffman 1915, cited in Goldsmith 1999, p. 189). In some primitive peoples arteriosclerosis, dental caries and cancers are so uncommon as to remain unnoticed (Dubos 1960, cited in Goldsmith 1999, p. 189). Such concerns about the real impact of health care on the health of societies suggest that the increasing scrutiny of the work of highly paid health professionals will continue to require greater vigilance of practice and better use of resources to maintain a relevant profile of effectiveness. In particular it can be expected that the ethics of health care resource use will be addressed more vigorously, with further creation of practice guidelines and standards (Nicholls et al 2000). Although such practice frameworks are possibly effective in rationalising care, their prescriptive nature can work against the innovation and discovery which could expand professional knowledge. The visibility of a profession's role in accountability and efficiency initiatives, both to maintain the respect of consumers and to attract newer generations, is vital. Use of networking and team working systems is important to strengthen the quality and improvement of interdisciplinary health care activities (Imanaka 1997).

Purchasing decisions are increasingly based on available evidence, despite critical analysis of the literature which shows not only an overall poor quality of studies but also a lack of studies generally, with some professions being grossly underrepresented, as examples of data synthesis systems such as the evidence-based medical database the Cochrane Library (www.update-software.com/cochrane) or the physiotherapy evidence database PEDRO (www.pedro.fhs.usyd.edu.au) can testify. If knowledge development is to progress on all fronts, the moral question arises of the necessity further to canvass awarding bodies to ensure an equity of support for all professions working in health care. In addition there is a need to address ethical concerns about withholding treatment in research studies where the intervention has yet to be proven. It is important to take a fresh look at the benefits of research on different treatment interventions with control groups within an inclusive holistic view of professional knowledge. It is necessary to provoke research funding groups to rethink their hierarchy of evidence that places knowledge generated via the sources we promulgate in this book at the bottom of the scale. Equally there is a need in times of limited funding to ensure that the arguments for 'blue-skies research which thinks the unthinkable' (Desforges 2001, p. 16) are persuasive. The quest for new knowledge that challenges accepted knowledge can be encouraged through lifelong learning practices in education (ibid., p. 23) and sustained through practice.

Can professional contributions to health match health care demands and develop practice knowledge further?

The match of the professions' contribution to health care needs is continually being examined as health care needs are re-evaluated. The growing availability of knowledge of the current scientific evidence base of practice, juxtaposed with management of health in small units where the information input can be based on power, can be seen to hail the end of clinical freedom. These changes in the focus of modern health care create the need for changes in the ways in which people currently work, which are often based on concepts of stable processes of health care and a linear system of referral patterns that have changed little over the years. The current attention to providing quality services for patients is changing the way health care is viewed. Some health systems, such as the UK National Health Service, have been built around an unspoken concept of sharing the economic risks of ill health from which patients have developed a sense of 'not wanting to jump the queue' if they perceive another patient to be more needy. Today an internal market that requires a costing of individual episodes of care inevitably exerts a pressure to discriminate against those at high risk (Eve & Hodgkin 1997, p. 81). This kind of assessment of the risks of future ill health for an individual can provide further opportunity to examine interaction processes between staff in the operationalisation of health care. Other outcomes of economic management can be quite the opposite. Some areas face the commodification of health (Neubauer 1998), where the cost of health care determines who can afford to purchase it and how much health the fund providers will designate as the fund member's entitlement.

Just as knowledge can be shaped by systems of work which constrain practice resources, so can consumers and stakeholders in health. Patient participation and user involvement are becoming more prevalent, as new ways of working take into account the multiple goals of varying stakeholders in health. Professional work should no longer be *on behalf of* but *with* patients, and should increasingly occur in purposeful interactions which are patient-led. However, this can lead to further shaping of practice activities in ways which can limit knowledge development. In a similar vein, the current world unrest prompts questions about consumers of a country's health resources. There are codes of conduct which call for an equity of care or which seek to delineate the parameters of that care. Such phenomena can increasingly confront our practice and may determine the limits of our commitment and identification with knowledge development in practice or determine our ability to pursue it. Expressing knowledge can be a source of effective practice or a source of delineation of practice (Sternberg 1999), and careful reflection is required to consider how knowledge is disclosed in each context.

A special competence is required for transdisciplinary work involving a merged approach to client-focused care (Gibbons et al 1999), in areas such as mental health, terminal illness care and pain management. True interdisciplinary work involves suspension of known methods and a focus on the problem (de Wachter 1982). Transdisciplinary work, whilst morally a high level of practice, creates a paradox of the need for specialist knowledge which then becomes merged with the knowledge of others, to create new knowledge that transcends disciplinary boundaries (Gibbons et al 1999). In these situations it is important to keep a clear focus on professional practice to ensure that the contribution to the common task solution is not ignored in the development of the knowledge of the individual profession.

How can changes in education affect the development of knowledge of practice?

Since 1988 the WHO has vigorously promoted learning together to work together (WHO 1988) as a means of cultivating collaboration between professionals in health and social care, and ultimately to enhance patient care (Zwarenstein et al 2002). The reality of health care practice has provided a major stimulus to interprofessional education aimed at improving patient care. But there are drawbacks to knowledge development for individual professions in shared learning and in shared knowledge situations (Wood 2001). Students entering any of the health care professions not only must acquire a large range of knowledge, skills and attitudes during their course, but must do this partly within learning environments where the principal activity is the delivery of health services. Much classroom teaching can appear remote from the students' goals on entering the course, which can be highly altruistic and profession-specific. It is not surprising that students develop strong academic and social support systems within their peer groups as part of the process of professional socialisation. These peer groups help to foster students' confidence in demonstrating their knowledge and skills, and help them to become aware of what is unique in their particular professional perspective. Learning in multidisciplinary contexts provides an opportunity to develop an awareness of different views of professional knowledge, prior to encountering other professions in the workplace after graduation.

Access to higher education is widening and further scrutiny of the professions will lead to a further need to demonstrate public accountability (Edwards & Higgs 1999, Morris 2002). In the UK, as in many European countries, there will be more state and public input into higher education decision-making. At present there is a call for membership of the health professions to reflect the demographics of the community, with representation of ethnic groups and ages (Morris 2002). Alongside this change has been a call for educational strategies that focus on competencies needed for decision-making and for participating in change (Hunt & Higgs 1999, Centre for the Advancement of Interprofessional Education 2002). Concepts of competence are socially and individually situated and can have a range of meanings (Eraut 1998). In the UK, for example, the Disability Discrimination Act 1995 has influenced thinking regarding the limits and discipline-specificity of competence in practice (Chartered Society of Physiotherapy 2001, 2002). A set of definitions relevant to education of health and social care practitioners and a consensus of representations of competence in professional models of practice are sought, but creative learning pathways will be needed to prepare professionals with enthusiasm and initiative (Eraut 1998). Knowledge development will be determined or constrained by the way in which the relationship between theory and practice is conceptualised and interpreted (ibid.).

How may increasing use of cyberspace influence development of professional knowledge?

Use of cyberspace favours those who can access it. Access to the internet is growing all over the world. A recent estimate (February 2001) suggests that there were '95 million Internet users in Europe by the end of 2000. Updated figures from December 2002 show Asia Pacific as the largest region of growth with 178 million Internet users in 2001, which will grow to over 615 million Internet users in 2007. Western Europe with 290 million Internet users in 2007 will also top the 230 million Internet users forecasted for the United States. The Middle East/Africa region will have the lowest number of Internet users at 96 million in 2007, but showing strong growth from 8 million Internet users in 1999' (http://www.etforecasts.com).

Use of the internet has several potential implications for the development of professional knowledge. One consequence of enhanced communications is that specialist knowledge today is less contained. It is socially distributed and is the preserve of neither university nor practice (Gibbons et al 1999). Knowledge located on global websites is continually being combined and recombined (ibid.). Through the internet, there is also a compression of time and space (Edwards & Usher 2000) which allows people in different locations to connect with each other much more quickly than ever before. Participation in online education challenges the traditional roles of students and teachers. Students' focus shifts from membership of an institution, which provides a sense of boundaries and clear expectations, to a new identity in which the student is 'an individualised, flexible and lifelong learner engaging in learning practice' (ibid., p. 126). In this new learning environment the choices available and the choice conditions shape situations of less certainty, and less stable identities. Instead of making postmodern society more transparent, the new media make it more complex and even chaotic. What was once the 'reality of the world' has now become a context of a 'multiplicity of fablings' (Deegan et al 1996, p. 8). We know little today of the impact of this communications revolution on the development of professional knowledge in students (Richardson & Cooper 2003) and how they manage the ever-increasing information coming from diverse sources. A clear sense of epistemological beliefs and self-regulatory skills (Hartley & Bendixen 2001) is needed to help learners to be selective if learning is to be effectively tailored to professional practice.

High-calibre graduates are creating a challenge for university systems. Universities are no longer monopoly suppliers of higher education; they face competition from national and international partnerships which can include researchers and clinicians (Gibbons et al 1999). If fully used, these partnerships can provide processes of creating networks of innovation and practice with universally global prospects of data analysis generating new knowledge. As an example, the SETI project (www.setiathome.ssl.berkeley.edu/), which uses home computers to search for extraterrestrial intelligence through analysis of huge data sets of astronomical radio noise from radio telescopes, will provide information that can be generated only through cyberspace and thus is integrally related to it.

New methods, new protocols and forms of assembling knowledge challenge how what we know relates to what we used to know or believed we knew. Questions are being raised about the status of authority and knowledge as shaped by the new electronic technologies (Deegan et al 1996). Libraries are less like storehouses and more like nodes in an information retrieval system (Pickering 1996). It is possible that change in the 'habitus' of academic culture, that is, the set of dispositions, tastes, practices and values that are developed, shared and transmitted by a community of practice, may place more significance on ownership of CD-ROMs and use of specific hypertext links than on books, signalling the profound impact of information technology on knowledge development.

SUMMARY

In this chapter we have reflected on many practice epistemology issues in the context of the health professions. We have addressed the questions: What do we know about the knowledge needed for health care? What would practice look like that is carried out by professionals who know about knowing? What more can be done to explain and characterise practice knowledge? What are some of the social trends and structures of practice that may influence further evolution of professional knowledge development? Key arguments presented include the importance of reflective practice, the value of peers and practice communities, the need to rethink research and the resulting knowledge for practice, the importance of understanding the nature of practice knowledge, the need to check continually whether professional knowledge is adequate for practice and community needs, the need to recognise the reciprocity between growth and change in practice and knowledge, and the importance of keeping in tune with the information technology revolution (as a tool for, not master of practice).

Readers, whether from a practice, education or research background, can consider the implications of these issues for their role as knowledge users and knowledge creators. More than ever the rapidly changing worlds of work and society are providing many challenges to the adequacy (in breadth and depth) of the knowledge bases of our professions and the capacity of our professionals to critique, refine and enlarge our knowledge to meet the needs of our stakeholders.

REFERENCES

Barach, P. & Moss, F. (2001). Delivering safe health care: safety is the patient's right and the obligation of all health professionals. *Quality in Health Care*, **10**, 199–203.

Bereiter, C. & Scardamalia, M. (1996). Re-thinking learning. In *The Handbook of Education and Human Development: New Models of Learning, Teaching and Schooling* (D. R. Olson & N. Torrance, eds) pp. 485–513. Cambridge, MA: Blackwell.

Bond, M. (2002). *An Investigation of Factors that Inhibit or Facilitate Access and Utilisation of Research Information by Therapy Professionals.* Unpublished PhD thesis. Norwich, UK: University of East Anglia.

Broadbent, J., Dietrich, M. & Roberts, J. (eds) (1997). *The End of Professions? The Restructuring of Professional Work.* London: Routledge.

Centre for the Advancement of Interprofessional Education (2002). *Higher Professional Education for Adapting to Change and for Participating in Managing Change on Behalf of Society as well as Within the Professions.* Report of the European Interprofessional Consultation 1999–2001. London: UK Centre for the Advancement of Interprofessional Education.

Chartered Society of Physiotherapy (2001). *CSP Duties under the Disability Discrimination Act.* London: Chartered Society of Physiotherapy.

Chartered Society of Physiotherapy (2002). *Abilitynet Myths and Realities – Awareness Raising and Practical Action.* London: Chartered Society of Physiotherapy.

Cochrane Library *www.update-software.com/cochrane/* (accessed 28 February 2003).

Deegan, M., Chernaik, W. & Gibson, A. (1996). Introduction. In *Beyond the Book: Theory, Culture and the Politics of Cyberspace* (W. Chernaik, M. Deegan & A. Gibson, eds) pp. 1–9. Oxford: Office for Humanities Communication, Humanities Computing Unit, Oxford University Computing Services.

Desforges, C. (2001). *Familiar Challenges and New Approaches: Necessary Advances in Theory and Methods in Research on Teaching and Learning.* The Desmond Nuttal/Carfax Memorial Lecture. Nottingham: British Educational Research Association.

de Wachter, M.A.M. (1982). Interdisciplinary bioethics: but where do we start? *Journal of Medicine and Philosophy*, **7**, 275–87.

Dubos, R. (1960). Introduction. In *Cancer: Disease of Civilisation? An Anthropological and Historical Study* (V. Stefansson, ed.) pp. ix–xi. New York: Hill and Wang.

Edwards, H. & Higgs, J. (1999). Challenges, cooperation and choice: creating the future of health professional education. In *Educating Beginning Practitioners: Challenges for Health Professional Education* (J. Higgs & H. Edwards, eds) pp. 289–96. Oxford: Butterworth-Heinemann.

Edwards, R. & Usher, R. (2000). *Globalisation and Pedagogy: Space, Place and Identity.* London: Routledge.

Eraut, M. (1998). Concepts of competence. *Journal of Interprofessional Care*, **12**(12), 127–39.

Eve, R. & Hodgkin, P. (1997). The restructuring of professional work. In *Professionalism and Medicine – the End of Professions?* (J. Broadbent, M. Dietrich & J. Roberts, eds) pp 69–85. London: Routledge.

Gibbons, M., Limoges, C., Nowotny, H. et al (1999). *The New Production of Knowledge: The Dynamics of Science and Research in Contemporary Societies.* London: Sage Publications.

Goldsmith, Z. (1999). Why globalisation is bad for your health. *The Ecologist*, **29**(3), 189–94.

Hartley, K. & Bendixen, L. D. (2001). Educational research in the internet age: examining the role of individual characteristics. *Educational Researcher*, **30**(9), 22–6.

Hoffman, F. L. (1915). *The Mortality from Cancer Throughout the World.* New York: The Prudential Press.

Hunt, A. & Higgs, J. (1999). Learning generic skills. In *Educating Beginning Practitioners: Challenges for Health Professional Education* (J. Higgs & H. Edwards, eds) pp. 166–72. Oxford: Butterworth-Heinemann.

Imanaka, Y. (1997). Professionalism and consumerism: can they grow together? *International Journal of Quality in Health Care*, **9**(6), 395–7.

Johnstone P. & Lacey, P. (2002). Are decisions by purchasers in an English health district evidence based? *Journal of Health Services Research*, **7**(3), 166–9.

Jones, M. & Higgs, J. (2000). Will evidence-based practice take the reasoning out of practice? In *Clinical Reasoning in the Health Professions*, 2nd edn (J. Higgs & M. Jones, eds) pp. 307–15. Oxford: Butterworth-Heinemann.

Morris, J. (2002). Current issues of accountability in physiotherapy and higher education: implications for physiotherapy educators. *Physiotherapy*, **88**(6), 354–63.

Nagel, E. (1961). *The Structure of Science: Problems in the Logic of Scientific Explanation*. London: Routledge & Kegan Paul.

Neubauer, D. (1998). *Impacts of Globalization on Health and Health Care Policy*. Occasional paper no. 1. Sydney: Centre for Professional Education Advancement, University of Sydney.

Nicholls, S., Cullen, R., O'Neill, S. & Halligan, A. (2000). Clinical governance, its origins and its foundations. *Clinical Performance and Quality Health Care*, **8**(3), 172–8.

PEDRO www.pedro.fhs.usyd.edu.au (accessed 28 February 2003).

Pickering, J. (1996). Hypermedia: when will they feel natural? In *Beyond the Book: Theory, Culture and the Politics of Cyberspace* (W. Chernaik, M. Deegan & A. Gibson, eds) pp. 43–53. Oxford: Office for Humanities Communication, Humanities Computing Unit, Oxford University Computing Services.

Richardson, B. & Cooper, N. (2003). Developing a virtual interdisciplinary research community in higher education. *Journal of Interprofessional Care*, **17**(2), 173–82.

Richardson, B., Lindquist, I., Engardt, M. & Aitman, C. (2002). Professional socialisation: students' expectations of being a physiotherapist. *Medical Teacher*, **24**(6), 622–7.

Schön, D. A. (1995). The new scholarship requires a new epistemology. *Change*, **27**(6), 26–34.

SETI www.setiathome.ssl.berkeley.edu/ (accessed 28 February 2003).

Sternberg, R. J. (1999). What do we know about tacit knowledge? Making the tacit become explicit. In *Tacit Knowledge in Professional Practice: Researcher and Practitioner Perspectives* (R. J. Sternberg & J. A. Horvath, eds) pp. 231–6. Mahwah, NJ: Lawrence Erlbaum Associates.

Titchen, A. (2000). *Professional Craft Knowledge in Patient-Centred Nursing and the Facilitation of its Development*. Oxford: Ashdale Press.

Tompson, M. M. & Ryan, A. G. (1996). The influence of fieldwork on the professional socialisation of occupational therapy students. *British Journal of Occupational Therapy*, **59**(2), 65–70.

Wilcock, P. M. (1998a). Never mind the quality: feel the improvement. *Quality in Health Care*, **7**, 181.

Wilcock, P. M. (1998b). The new NHS: an opportunity for modern, dependable thinking about quality improvement? *Healthcare Quality*, **4**(1–2), 21–5.

Windelband, W. (1915). Geschichte und Naturwissenschaft. In *Praeludien*, vol. 2, pp. 136–60. Tuebingen: J C B Mohr.

Wood, D. F. (2001). Interprofessional education – still more questions than answers. *Medical Education*, **35**, 816–17.

World Health Organization (1988). *Learning Together to Work Together for Health*. Geneva: WHO.

World Health Organization (2001). *International Classification of Functioning, Disability and Health*. Geneva: WHO.

Zwarenstein, M., Reeves, S., Barr, H. et al (2002). *Interprofessional Education: Effects on Professional Practice and Health Care Outcomes* (*Cochrane Review*). The Cochrane Library, issue 3, 2002. Oxford: Update Software.

Index

D